TUDOR CHILDBIRTH *in the* ROYAL COURT

To my husband Gordon for always believing in me, and in memory of Doctor Michel Odent who taught me the art of midwifery.

TUDOR CHILDBIRTH *in the* ROYAL COURT

THE MIDWIVES *and* MOTHERS

BRIGITTE BARNARD

PEN & SWORD HISTORY
AN IMPRINT OF PEN & SWORD BOOKS LTD.
YORKSHIRE – PHILADELPHIA

First published in Great Britain in 2026 by
PEN AND SWORD HISTORY
An imprint of
Pen & Sword Books Ltd
Yorkshire – Philadelphia

Print ISBN 978 1 03614 292 6
ePUB ISBN 978 1 03614 294 0
ePDF ISBN 978 1 03614 296 4

A CIP catalogue record for this book is available from the British Library.

Typeset in Times New Roman 11.5/14 by
SJmagic DESIGN SERVICES, India.
Printed and bound in the UK by CPI Group (UK) Ltd.

The Publisher's authorised representative in the EU for product safety is Authorised Rep Compliance Ltd., Ground Floor, 71 Lower Baggot Street, Dublin D02 P593, Ireland.
www.arccompliance.com

For a complete list of Pen & Sword titles please contact
PEN & SWORD BOOKS LIMITED
George House, Units 12 & 13, Beevor Street, Off Pontefract Road,
Barnsley, South Yorkshire, S71 1HN, England
E-mail: enquiries@pen-and-sword.co.uk
Website: www.pen-and-sword.co.uk

or

PEN AND SWORD BOOKS
1950 Lawrence Rd, Havertown, PA 19083, USA
E-mail: uspen-and-sword@casematepublishers.com
Website: www.penandswordbooks.com

FSC
www.fsc.org
MIX
Paper | Supporting responsible forestry
FSC® C013604

Contents

Acknowledgements

I would like to thank my dear friend, Wendy J. Dunn, for suggesting the idea for this book, and to the amazing staff at Pen and Sword Press, especially my editor Sarah Hodder, who has the patience of a saint, and to Sarah-Beth Watkins who encouraged me along the way. Midwives know that birth is not a single moment, but a process sometimes stalled by false starts, exhaustion, fear and resolve. Writing this book followed a similar rhythm. There were hours of silence when nothing happened then suddenly, progress! It was a remarkable journey, a labour of love and ultimately a good outcome. What more could a midwife want?

I would like to thank my four stoic children for their patience in enduring an admittedly short-tempered mother who often neglected getting their dinners done on time. Fortunately, they all seem to have survived the writing of this book. Thank you to the readers who will find in these pages a history of women who have seldom been acknowledged, the midwives who delivered some of England's greatest monarchs.

Introduction

Childbirth in the Tudor Age

In the shadowy and perfidious chambers of the Tudor court, power was made within the wombs of its queens. However ruthless, a kingdom rose and fell by its fecundity. A queen's worth was measured by a single unrelenting quantifier, her ability to provide the king with a healthy male child. With a midwife's trained eye, I have spent the past decade looking over historical accounts of the Tudors and their strange gynaecological history. The rise and fall of this dynasty – and its very survival – rested on a woman's ability to birth the succession. The delicate fronds of fallopian tubes and the cyclical waxing and waning of a royal womb and its skill for nourishing a foetus would ultimately decide the fate of an entire nation. The bedchamber was not just a sanctuary of intimacy; it was a high-stakes realm of dynastic achievement. The hope of the kingdom were sons, ideally three or more, as infant survival in the late Middle Age was hardly a given. The singular duty of a royal consort was to give the king a son; her triumph in the birthing chamber would ensure the continuation of the dynasty. Without a male heir, the succession teetered on the edge of chaos and made it vulnerable to the ruthless machinations of rival claimants. Pregnancy and childbirth were public spectacles of which a success secured a legacy; and failure met with disgrace, annulment, and even death. No family in history was more indelibly shaped by the drama of childbirth than the Tudors. The dynasty's dubious foundation rested on the survival of a single baby boy – Henry Tudor – who would become Henry VII. His formidable mother, Margaret Beaufort, would shape the nascent Tudor dynasty by sheer force of her will. Margaret gave birth to Henry Tudor in the damp, frosty isolation of Pembroke Castle on January 28, 1457. It was not simply a personal trial; it was the genesis of a dynasty irrespective of how difficult the event may or may not have been. Margaret birthed a son as well as a lineage that would one day grapple with reproductive strife for over a century. Her birth on that cold winter's day set the stage for a dynasty that would ultimately never win the war of successful reproductive strategy.

Childbirth in Tudor England was a whirlwind of significance, a personal triumph, communal event, and cultural cornerstone all at once. From the royal court to the rural cottages, it was steeped in rituals that walked a tightrope of hope, fear and superstition. Spiritually, childbirth was a sacred thing; the Tudors saw it as God's handiwork – a test of divine favour, where successes signalled blessings and loss was seen as a punishment. This blend of the practical and divine made childbirth a cultural linchpin, reflecting the Tudors' obsession with faith, lineage and survival. Having babies in the Tudor court was about securing power as well as posterity for royal women like Margaret Beaufort. For her, giving birth was a physical and political event that merged together a dynastic act, a personal sacrifice, and regal destiny.

When labour began, midwives would be summoned; queens as well as peasants relied upon them. These women would appear day or night ready to aid the labouring mother. Besides their profound knowledge they would be equipped with a bag of supplies, including herbs for speeding up labour, staunching bleeding, drying up the navel cord, easing labour pains and oils which were applied to the perineum, to mitigate tearing during birth. Midwives could manipulate the child's position within the womb to turn a poorly positioned baby, apply salves to ease straining muscles, and guide mothers through exhaustion.

If all went well, the room erupted in sounds of triumph. The baby was cleaned and swaddled tightly, the umbilical cord tied with a thread (sometimes kept as a keepsake), and handed to the mother or one of her ladies to admire. But success was never guaranteed – complications could snatch victory away in an instant, leaving the midwife to console the devastated mother. Under these tragic circumstances, the midwife's role turned solemn. If a baby was stillborn or fading fast, she'd baptise it on the spot, using a simple phrase: 'I christen thee in the name of the Father, the Son, and the Holy Ghost'. This baptism was often accomplished with a splash of water from a nearby bowl. It was a midwife's sacred duty, ensuring the infant's soul wasn't lost to limbo, according to the Catholic beliefs of the time. It's a reminder of how childbirth straddled the line between life and death.[1]

The Tudors marked childbirth with a trio of rituals. First came the queen's lying-in ceremony, then baptism, and finally the churching ceremony which reintroduced the queen back into public life amongst the court. The 'churching' ceremony occurred usually a month after birth. It was a rite of purification and gratitude, rooted in the New Testament tale of Mary presenting Jesus at the temple. The mother, veiled and escorted by her ladies-in-waiting, knelt at the church door while a priest recited psalms – often Psalm 121, 'I will lift up mine eyes unto the hills'. Then the woman would offer up a coin or a candle to complete the churching service. The new mother was traditionally accompanied by her female family members and friends. Then, the party! Wealth dictated the scale – royalty and members of the peerage would host grand banquets with several rich courses, while peasants shared ale and bread, and a 'groaning cheese', a wheel sliced only after birth, and 'groaning cake', passed around to honour the mother's success in childbirth.

Not every birth ended in celebration, however. Stillbirths and early losses were achingly common. A mother's death might prompt a 'cradle toll' – a slow bell to signal her passing while a child's loss was mourned with tiny shrouds and quick burials. The parent's community would offer food and prayers, showing solidarity in grief.[2]

The many customs around childbirth show a culture that met life's fragility with rituals to comfort, viewing every birth as a gift and a gamble. For royalty, this gambit reached its fevered peak in the reign of Henry VIII, a king whose obsession with securing a male heir upended his entire realm. Henry's desperate quest for a son drove him to marry six different women and to sever England's ties with Rome. Ultimately, Henry had to create his own religion in order to satisfy his desperate ambition for a son. Henry experienced loss after loss after loss, his first two wives suffering through numerous miscarriages or stillborn children. His first wife, Katherine of Aragon, suffered heartbreaking successions of miscarriages, stillbirths, and short-lived infants producing only one surviving child, a daughter. Unsatisfied with this outcome, Henry divorced Katherine and married Anne Boelyn. Tragically, Anne also failed to give the king a son; her first birth resulted in a daughter they named Elizabeth. Anne's subsequent pregnancies ended in a series of miscarriages, sealing her fate with a French swordsman's lethal arc. Henry married for a third time to Jane Seymour, who finally gave the king his golden prince. Henry's triumph turned to sorrow when his third wife mysteriously died ten days after Prince Edward's birth.

The question lingers, tantalising and unresolved – why did so many Tudor pregnancies end in sorrow? What unforeseen forces conspired to snuff out the lives of babes within the royal womb? The historical records offer no definitive answers, yet it teases us with clues of familial frailty, and decades of failed reproductive designs. The boys born of this dynastic line all died early deaths. Frailty stalks the descendants, but why? I shall venture forth into this enigma; weaving together a tapestry of evidence to propose compelling theories through the lens of modern medicine. I will closely examine the reproductive failures that plagued the Tudor queens using my extensive knowledge of childbirth; illuminating the mysteries of their suffering with insights that were unavailable to their physicians. First, let's shift our focus to the customs surrounding these births that created the royal lineage and explore how they were shaped in part by the formidable influence of Margaret Beaufort. Let's navigate the perilous terrain of dynastic childbirth.

Tudor Family Tree

House of Tudor (1400–1603)

Owen Tudor
(*c*.1400–1461)
m. Catherine of Valois (widow of Henry V)

↓

- Edmund Tudor
  Earl of Richmond
  ↓
  Henry Tudor (1457–1509)
  → Became Henry VII, King of England (1485–1509)
  m. Elizabeth of York (uniting Lancaster and York)
- Jasper Tudor
  Duke of Bedford
  (no legitimate issue)

Children of Henry VII and Elizabeth of York:

- Arthur
  (1486–1502)
  (died young)
  no issue
- Margaret
  (1489–1541)
  ↓
  m. James IV of Scotland
  King of England
  ↓
  James V of Scotland
  ↓
  Mary, Queen of Scots (1542–1587)
  m. Henry Stuart, Lord Darnley
  ↓
  James VI of Scotland (1566–1625)
  Became James I of England in 1603
  (Start of House of Stuart in England)
- Henry VIII
  (1491–1547)
- Mary Tudor
  (1496–1533)
  m. (1) Louis XII of France
  (2) Charles Brandon,
  Duke of Suffolk
- Others

Children of Henry VIII:

- Mary I
  (1516–1558)
  Queen 1553–1558
  no surviving issue
- Elizabeth I
  (1533–1603)
  Queen 1558–1603
  no issue
- Edward VI
  (1537–1553)
  King 1547–1553
  no issue
- Others
  (died in infancy)

Mary Tudor (younger) branch (via Charles Brandon)
↓
Frances Brandon
↓
Lady Jane Grey (1537–1554)
'Nine Days' Queen' 1553 → executed, no issue

Part 1
Mothers of the Crown

Chapter 1

Mother of Destiny: Margaret Beaufort

Lady Margaret lays her weary, sweat-soaked head on the goose down pillow. Her large eyes are smudged with dark circles, enhancing her extreme youth and her pale, piquant little face. 'You have a fine son, your Grace, a big, healthy boy!' The midwife lifts up the red bawling newborn for Margaret to see.

'Jesu be praised! My husband would have been so pleased', the young woman replies in a ragged voice. She does not ask to hold the child. The midwife attends to the infant while a servant gives Margaret a cup of ale which the new mother drinks thirstily. The midwife is soon back with the small, squirming bundle. Margaret waves her away and says, 'He should be taken to the wet nurse. I will look upon him anon, after I have rested'. The midwife curtseys and steps out of the birthing chamber while her assistant helps to make the young woman comfortable. Margaret Beaufort is soon sound asleep, her body making only a little bump under the many luxurious comforters.

Before the Tudors, England was engulfed in one of the bloodiest civil wars in its history – the Wars of the Roses (1455-1487). On one side were the Lancastrians whose symbol was the red rose, and on the other were their cousins, the Plantagenets or House of York, symbolised by the white rose. At its core, this war was about the struggle for the English throne with each faction declaring themselves to have a stronger claim to the monarchy. For thirty years the crown changed hands multiple times with kings being overthrown, murdered, imprisoned or killed in battle. The war concluded with the rise of Henry Tudor (Henry VII) whose mother, Margaret Beaufort, was from the Lancastrian side and his wife, Elizabeth of York, from the Plantagenets. Thus was born the Tudor rose, a rose with a white centre and outer petals of red displaying the successful merging of the rival factions and ending the Wars of the Roses. Yet Henry Tudor's ascension to the throne was far from certain. His claim was weak and his survival dependent upon the resilience and extraordinary determination of one woman – his mother Margaret.

Margaret Beaufort was born in the spring of 1443 at Bletsoe near Higham Ferrers, the patrimonial estate of her mother. Margaret's family was a noble but politically fragile family. She was the only daughter of Margaret Beauchamp and the Earl of Somerset.

Somerset would later commit suicide after a disastrous campaign led by him against France in 1443. Margaret must have learned as a young child how to overcome adversity; her family's reputation would have been severely tarnished as suicide was considered a mortal sin in the Catholic Church. Her father's death left her the heiress of a vast fortune in the form of lands – her father had property in Kent, Worcestershire, Lincolnshire, Norfolk, Somerset, Essex and Sussex. A girl with wealth and royal blood would later make her a very precious and highly sought-after commodity on the marriage market.[3]

Margaret received an excellent education; she learned Latin and to speak fluent French. She was exceptionally intelligent and was well-read – her love of books becoming a lifelong passion. Margaret was also an extremely devout Catholic and was extolled for her piety by her peers later in her life. Young Margaret also had an interest in medicinals and healing; she loved learning about herb craft and spent a portion of each day attending to the needs of the lower class wounded or sick in her community. She would ask an ill person about their symptoms and provide them with whatever herbal remedy she thought would best improve their malady. She viewed this care of the poor as part of her Christian duty.[4]

When Margaret was still a very young girl, she was given as a ward to William de la Pole, Earl of Suffolk. At the age of 7, she entered into a marriage with the earl's son, John de la Pole, who was 8 years old at the time. The marriage was a verbal contract only, given the fact that the bride and groom were so very young. The relationship never became what most would consider a real marriage in the true sense of the word.

William de la Pole did himself no favours by joining together his son with the wealthy and noble Margaret Beaufort because a few months later he was impeached by parliament who suspected he sought the English crown through Margaret's royal lineage, should King Henry VI die without issue. Suffolk was banished to Calais where he was executed and his body thrown into the sea. When his body eventually washed up onto the shores of Dover, his remains were taken back to England where he received a proper burial at the Church of Saint Andrew at Wingfield, Suffolk.

The disgrace and murder of William de la Pole had little to no effect on Margaret, it's even possible that the two had never even met.

Now that Margaret was no longer a ward, she was one of England's wealthiest landowners, so it's no surprise that many were interested in what would become of her now. Margaret and her mother were invited to court in February 1443 to appear before King Henry VI. Henry summoned the girl to appear before him and must have been pleased by what he saw because he wasted no time in having her so-called marriage to John de la Pole annulled in order to marry young Margaret to his half-brother, Edmund Tudor. Margaret was said to have been visited by Saint Nicholas one evening as she contemplated the proposed marriage to Edmund; 'whether sleeping or waking she could not assure, but about 4 of ye clock, one appeared unto her arrayed like a bishop and naming unto her Edmond [*sic*], take him unto her husband'.[5]

This story helped Margaret to create a special visionary mystique about herself that conveyed an aura of spiritual purity, raising her far above other mortals in her closeness to God. It also demonstrated that her union with Edmund Tudor was a divinely ordained marriage that would lead to a grand destiny. Margaret's religious fervour was said to have been so fanatical that each day she would kneel before her sacred icons, pressing her forehead to the cold stone floor in fervent prostration. Faith was not merely a part of her life, it consumed her, shaping her every thought and ambition. Her confessor claimed that Margaret had a fancy to 'rescue the Holy Land away from the Infidels; her enthusiastic ardour almost amounted to fanaticism but was tempered with so much humility that she would often say that if the princes of Christendom would combine and march against the Turks, she would willingly attend the camp in some menial way'.[6]

Margaret Beaufort's piety was more than mere devotion. It was the unwavering conviction that she had been singled out by God for a divine purpose … her prayers were not just acts of faith, but declarations of her own sanctity; each whispered supplication reinforcing the belief that she was set apart, chosen. In her mind, she was not simply a servant of God, but a vessel of his will. Her suffering, a mark of holiness, her ambition, a righteous calling.

Margaret benefited from her newly acquired proximity to the Crown, and her husband Edmund now had all of Margaret's land bequeathed to him. Nine days after she turned 12, Margaret went to live with Edmund at Pembrokeshire in southern Wales where they took up residence at the Palace of Lamphey. She was now styled the Countess of Richmond and became to her husband Edmund a wife in every sense of the word. Descriptions of Margaret paint a picture of a very small, slender child, hardly ready to perform her duties in the marital bed. The Catholic Church decreed that a girl of 12 was old enough to wed and to consummate the marriage, although this was not the standard of the era. Most of Margaret's contemporaries considered 12 too young for intercourse and married youth would wait several more years before consummating the marriage. Edmond Tudor's 'reckless disregard for Margaret's physical underdevelopment would leave her with deep emotional and possibly physical scars'.[7]

In no time at all, Margaret was pregnant, at barely 13 years of age. Her husband, meanwhile, was engaged in a battle with Gruffud ap Nicholas whose pride was pricked by the presence of a man more well connected than himself. In August of 1456, Edmund Tudor took over the impressive stone keep of Carmarthen Castle, a stronghold in that area of Wales and the apple of Richard of York's eye. York did not take kindly to a Lancastrian stalwart occupying his castle, so he assembled an army and confronted Edmund Tudor. On 10 August, York had taken back his castle and thrown Edmund in prison. Although Edmund was released, he died of the plague on 1 November at Carmarthen Castle. At this point, 13-year-old Margaret was seven months pregnant and she was all alone in plague-infested Wales.

Jasper Tudor, Margaret's brother-in-law, arrived and brought the heavily pregnant girl to Pembroke Castle sometime in mid to late November. On January 28, Margaret successfully delivered a baby boy whom she would name Henry. Margaret would have had a midwife-attended birth, but no records exist describing the labour. Margaret probably suffered in her long and lonely labour without her mother or even any friends present for emotional support.

In terms of the birth itself, the only known complication was Margaret's stunted growth. Girls will not continue to grow after giving birth which might explain Margaret's well documented short stature.[8]

Bishop Fisher was known to have said, 'like Moses [Henry] was wonderfully born and brought into this world by his noble princess mother, who was very small of stature as she was never a tall woman. It seemed a miracle that, and at that age and so little a personage, anyone should have been born at all, let alone one so tall and fine of build as her son'.[9]

Nicola Tallis describes the birth as physically and psychologically traumatic and that it caused Margaret Beaufort permanent damage which rendered her infertile.[10] Elizabeth Norton likewise describes Margaret's birth: 'Margaret suffered considerably during the birth of her only child. It's been suggested that the birth caused permanent damage to her body'.[11] No contemporary sources describe Margaret's birth as difficult. Margaret herself never said or wrote anything about her childbirth being unusually traumatic, and no other primary source mentions it. In fact, she celebrated the day she gave birth to her son with tremendous joy. As a midwife who has worked with many teenage girls, I found them to be remarkably resilient and able to bounce back after childbirth with remarkable speed. Margaret was 13 years and 8 months old when she gave birth to Henry. While this is quite young, I found several other instances in the fifteenth and sixteenth centuries of girls around the same age as Margaret who had successful pregnancies and births with no subsequent infertility issues. Very young women may have children without complications. The few who did have problems were the same issues that could also affect older women – puerperal fever and haemorrhage being among the causes. Some historians assume that Margaret's lack of further pregnancies demonstrates that her first birth damaged her in some way. There is no proof for this assumption, perhaps the cause lay with her husbands or for some other reason.

Margaret would never conceive another child again though she married twice more. What is written in the historical records of the time points to the possibility that Margaret suffered from her early experiences of sexual intercourse at the age of 12. When her own granddaughter Margaret became engaged to James IV, she beseeched her son not to let the young Margaret marry too early lest James 'injure her and endanger her health' in his eagerness to bed his young bride. Dyspareunia and spasms of the vagina are common problems experienced by women who have had traumatic sexual experiences in childhood.[12] If Margaret experienced such symptoms, intercourse may have become impossible for her to endure. It is known that Margaret would later undertake a formal vow of celibacy renouncing sexual intimacy forevermore, indicating that she disliked it intensely.

Shortly after giving birth to her son Henry, Margaret Beaufort returned to her estates in Lincolnshire. She would not see her son again for nearly fourteen years. It seemed as if young Margaret did not have any particular desire to raise her baby boy herself, on the contrary, she seemed very happy to leave her child behind in the care of servants at Pembroke Castle. Young Henry would later become the ward of Sir William Herbert, in 1461, and Margaret was content to have very little to do with motherhood. On January 3, 1458, Margaret married for a third time, to Henry Stafford. Margaret was now called Lady Stafford, and together with her new husband she took up residence at Woking Palace in Surrey. Margaret's marriage to Stafford marked the beginning of a quieter phase of her life before she began her relentless efforts to secure her son's ascension to the English throne. They resided primarily at Woking Palace at Surrey. The couple initially avoided direct involvement in the Cousin's War which by 1455 had the Lancastrian king Henry VI pitted against the York claimant, Richard Duke of York.[13]

Margaret's relatively calm life was about to implode in 1461 when Edward, Earl of March, the son of Richard, Duke of York, seized the throne, deposing the weak king Henry VI and becoming Edward IV. Lancastrian stalwarts like Margaret and her husband were forced into submission or exile. Young Henry Tudor became a more prominent figure in this shifting landscape as one of the only remaining Lancastrians who had any claim to the title of king.

Unable to remain neutral, Margaret and Henry Stafford stayed loyal to the red rose of Lancaster. Margaret's husband entered the fray and went to battle for the Lancastrian side in 1472 during the Battle of Barnet, where he was grievously wounded. Stafford died later that year leaving Margaret a widow for the third time at the age of 28.[14]

At this point, Henry Tudor was a youth of 14 when his uncle Jasper took him to Brittany, out of the reach of his Yorkist enemies. Although Margaret was not a doting mother, she was satisfied to see her son safely out of harm's way, Margaret's thoughts then turned to her own safety. She needed to find a man with power and position who would help her navigate the treacherous waters of the political climate. Her choice landed on Thomas Stanley, who had ties to both York and Lancaster. Now Margaret could bide her time, and plan her son's return to England. Stanley's clever duplicity kept them safe during Edward IV's reign.[15]

Margaret cultivated allies and remained in contact with her son and Jasper through letters during this new phase of her life. She gave generously to Catholic charities and religious houses, building up her legacy as a pious Christian and possibly obfuscating her political ambitions for her son. Meanwhile, Jasper Tudor turned young Henry into a capable fighter as well as an astute politician during this time where there were very few Lancastrian heirs to be found.[16]

In 1483 England underwent another political earthquake when Edward IV died. His 12-year-old son briefly succeeded him but disappeared before his coronation along with his little brother Richard, Duke of York. The man who then became king of England was Edward IV's brother, Richard, now King Richard III. Margaret began working on her own son's claim to the throne in what was known as Buckingham's Rebellion. The rebellion failed and Margaret was put under house arrest, with her husband Stanley charged with keeping her subdued under lock and key.

Margaret had other ideas, however, and she intensified her efforts to gain the crown for her son. She negotiated with Elizabeth Woodville, Edward IV's widow, to betroth her eldest daughter, Elizabeth of York, to Henry Tudor; an ingenious plan that would merge together the rival factions of Lancaster and York and once and for all to end the Cousin's War. Elizabeth Woodville agreed and in 1485 the time had come. Margaret had raised funds and secured promises of fealty from alienated noblemen including ones in France where Henry was sheltered after fleeing Brittany. At the Battle of Bosworth Field on August 22 1485, Richard III faced Henry Tudor's army. Stanley and his brother held back their armies until the very last moment, then rode in and helped Henry to defeat Richard, making Henry king due to his victory on the battlefield.[17]

On October 30, 1485, Henry Tudor was crowned king at Westminster Abbey, fulfilling his mother's ambitions for him. Margaret created a new title for herself, 'My Lady, The King's Mother'. From that day forward she signed her letters Margaret R; presumably 'R' for Regina or queen. A new dynasty was born and Margaret was prepared to codify the customs for the new court, shaping it to her liking.[18]

Margaret had a personality moulded by adversity and knowing how to best overcome it. She was incredibly resourceful and resilient, qualities she honed from a very young age. She had a single-minded determination and drive. Undoubtedly, Margaret was extremely pious, and she cultivated an almost saintly mystique about herself which she probably felt gave nearly divine credence to her decisions. Margaret had a good deal of pragmatism in her personality too, and could be ruthless if necessary. Her traits of resilience, piety, authority, pragmatism and meticulousness were the necessary qualities one would need to set forth new court protocols. The Tudor court, emerging from the chaos of the thirty-years-long Wars of the Roses, required a new framework to assert itself. Margaret transformed the Tudor court into a structured, symbolically rich institution that reinforced Tudor legitimacy and stability.[19]

Chapter 2

Childbirth Practices and Protocols of the Tudor Court

Margaret Beaufort's personality was the crucible in which key Tudor court customs were forged. By codifying childbirth rituals, and assuring maternal precedence, she shaped the court into a bastion of royal legitimacy. Her legacy as a protocol-shaper underscores her importance as not only the king's mother but also as a visionary who imprinted her character onto an era. The childbirth rituals of the Tudor court were created by Margaret Beaufort partly as a reaction to her own childbirth experience. Her son's birth had been endured privately in a cold and drafty stone castle far away from either friend or family. Margaret was determined to see that royal women never again had to suffer a birth like her own. Margaret sought to emphasise the dynastic importance of childbirth, and also to ensure the comfort, safety and aesthetic surroundings for the pregnant queen.

Margaret started writing her Ordinances in 1486 when her daughter-in-law, Elizabeth of York, was pregnant with her first child, Arthur. The protocols had remarkable detail, down to the number and colour of the cushions that should be used to decorate the confinement chambers. Drawing from the 1493 Household Ordinances – documents regulating court life – as well as her own life experiences, Margaret established a meticulous protocol that emphasised seclusion, ritual purity and royal spectacle. Royal childbirth must happen in the most luxurious setting possible, with every conceivable comfort provided for the queen before she even stepped one well-shod foot into her confinement chamber.[20]

Four to six weeks before the expected date of childbirth, the queen would 'take to her chambers'. Margaret choreographed the spectacle down to the smallest detail. First came the Mass beseeching the Almighty for heavenly benevolence. Then the queen, dressed in sumptuous velvets or silks and bedecked in jewels, her belly proudly thrust forward, walked slowly past the courtiers lined up on either side of the route to the confinement chambers. The queen brought with her a select group of her ladies-in-waiting and female members of her family which might include her mother, sisters, or cousins. A priest was at hand bearing a missal and musicians played an appropriate piece of music for the occasion. The court ladies carried candles or bouquets of rosemary – a token of fidelity and remembrance. Then the king would give his wife a blessing and perhaps a gift, then finally the priest would bless the queen and hand her a psalter or other religious token. Then the queen would cross over the threshold of her chambers with her women, and the door would close, sealing her off from the rest of the world until after her child was born and she had recovered from the birth. This moment was orchestrated by Margaret to build anticipation that would climax with the triumphant birth of the heir.[21]

Inside the confinement chambers, the walls and windows were covered with beautiful Arras tapestries depicting serene scenes from the bible – nothing violent for that was thought to be harmful to the mother and the child within her womb. Darkness was deemed necessary by Margaret Beaufort to shield the precious inhabitants from evil spirits as well as to preserve the mother's 'delicate' eyesight. Draughts and fresh air were considered unhealthy for the tender newborn and was eschewed in the birthing chamber. Dozens of candles illuminated the rooms and besides the richly draped tester bed, a huge pallet bed for the queen to use during labour was placed in the centre of the room dressed in crimson satin. Everything in the confinement room was decorated in shades of red and gold. Flanking either side of the pallet were the cradles; one made of wood for practical use and one very elaborate and highly decorative solid silver one for State ceremony. Cupboard doors were open to display gold plate as well as wine, food, and spices. Margaret's list of items for the confinement chambers was exacting; she lists linen from Rheims, Tartian silk, fine lawn and wool, fustian pillows stuffed with down, furred panels, head sheets, and the list goes on.[22]

Daily deliveries of fresh food and beverages ensured that the queen and her women didn't have to concern themselves with such mundane matters as sustenance. The queen's midwife was at her beck and call but did not dwell within the confinement room with the queen. The daily care of the queen fell to her women, and the midwife made an appearance on an as-needed basis. No men were permitted inside the queen's lying-in chambers with the exception of a priest to hold private services for the queen and her women. The queen whiled away her days with her ladies or 'gossips' as they were often called, talking, playing cards, reading aloud and listening to musicians play (probably outside the queen's chamber).

When the hour of the birth was at hand the queen's midwives took over. Young, unmarried women were not thought fit to witness the labour and birth and were ushered out of the birthing chamber. The remaining ladies helped to make the queen comfortable during the first stage of labour, taking turns walking with her and encouraging her during painful contractions.

There is a common misconception that midwives employed bizarre and possibly dangerous methods in their craft. 'Historical writing about midwives has sometimes been sensationally misguided.'[23] This is a result of reading only select instances that are truly unique and strange but is not a factual representation of midwifery in the Tudor or any age. Midwives practiced in the sixteenth century in many ways exactly as modern homebirth midwives practice today. They were highly competent and well-respected women who were either married or widowed, and they were not dirty, incompetent, superstitious fools raving about evil spirits in the birthing chamber. Superstitions were part of the culture in the late medieval era, but this was not a trait reserved for birthing attendants. If anything, midwives were less superstitious and more down-to-earth than most of their peers due to their close connection to the everyday miracle of childbirth. The denigration of midwives is likely due to the genesis of obstetrics and the introduction of male doctors in a previously female only sphere beginning in the late seventeenth century. At this time of transition from female midwives to male accoucheurs, the rates of neonatal and maternal deaths went up, not down. Once male-led obstetrics became popular the statistics post 1700–1900 climbed to as high as 30 per cent, as opposed to the rates of 1-2 per cent in the sixteenth century midwifery-led period. Then when women started giving birth in hospitals attended by obstetricians in the decades before hygiene, the deaths went up to 20–30 per cent, often due to cadaver particles. At that time doctors didn't understand why delivering a baby after dissecting a cadaver was a dangerous practice. It was the discovery of handwashing combined with antibiotics that was responsible for turning around high maternal deaths.[24]

It's time to put to bed the myth of the Tudor age midwife and her superstitious and 'dangerous practices'. These were competent women who took their practice very seriously. It's unfortunate that some historians have taken the strangest anecdotes found in medieval texts and used these instances as evidence that all midwives practiced like ignorant fools. Tudor age women fared well in childbirth despite the perception that they perished in droves. The odds of survival were very good for women barring any unusual circumstances in the Tudor age.

The sixteenth century was a superstitious era and some of that superstition naturally found its way into the birthing chamber. Many of the Tudor queens were granted 'holy relics' to give them succour and something to focus on during labour. These relics could be girdles said to have been worn by the Virgin Mary or an icon. Nesting stones, while not religious relics, were also a commonly seen item in the hands of a labouring woman. These stones supposedly came from Cyprus or Africa and their powers were generated by the principles of sympathies. The stone within the stone symbolised the safety of the infant within the royal womb. It was thought to be prudent to loosen all fastenings and untie any ribbons, in order to allow the labour to progress unencumbered.[25]

The midwives would have stood back observing the pace of the labour, allowing the queen the freedom to do as her body commanded. If the first stage dragged on too long the midwife might have given the queen a concoction of labour stimulating herbs such as pennyroyal, galbanum resin, motherwort, mugwort or rue. These herbs could be very potent and would have been used with considerable caution. Another method of helping a sluggish labour along would have been to check the baby's position in the womb; if a head was not firmly pressing down on the mouth of the womb, the contractions would not serve to open the cervix. A small adjustment made to the infant's head could rapidly change the speed of labour. Many readers will be surprised by what I am going to say now – a breech baby would not pose a problem as long as the presenting part was the child's buttocks. A bottom serves to dilate the cervix in the same way the head does. As long as the baby's head is flexed down with the chin toward the chest, the delivery is straightforward.

Unusual presentations like a footling breech or a transverse lie would have been repositioned long before the start of labour by the midwife, unless the child refused to be moved in which case there would be a significant chance of a bad outcome. These situations were uncommon but very problematic.

Once the moment of transition was at hand the midwife may have encouraged her client to sit upon the birthing stool, but moving a woman in this stage of labour is easier said than done. Positions for labour would have included hands-and-knees or on 'all fours', side-lying with the upper leg supported by the attending midwife, or she would be sat down upon the aforementioned stool. Oil may have been applied to the perineum to ease the head out. Immediately following the birth, one midwife would clear the infant's breathing passages by applying suction with her own mouth while the other midwife attended to the mother's needs. A lady-in-waiting would inform the Lord Great Chamberlain of the birth who would then inform the king.

Then the cord would be tied with thread and cut with the midwife's knife; a tool used specifically for this purpose. I discovered many interesting pieces of superstition around the navel cord such as, 'If it [the cord] have any wrinkles in it, then so many children shall the woman have in time to come'. Likewise, many believed that carrying a piece of the string would keep them safe from disease.[26]

After tying up and cutting the umbilical cord, the midwife would deliver the placenta. The placenta would be examined carefully by the midwives for any missing pieces and then put aside to be buried later. Then the midwives would clean the baby with anything from milk mixed with warm water to wine. Even butter could be used to clean a newborn baby. Then the swaddling bands were wrapped around the baby, and the royal child was dressed in fine clothing. Finally, the infant would receive a sprinkle of salt and a cross traced over it before a coin was placed in its cradle or hand.[27]

While the midwives were attending to the newborn baby, the queen's women would help her to have a sponge bath and get dressed in a fresh nightgown. Linen towels would be placed between her legs, held in place with a sling and tied around the queen's hips below her abdomen. Her hair would be brushed and arranged, and she was now helped into her richly appointed State bed supported by bolsters and many pillows. Once she was clean and presentable the king came to visit his new baby and the queen. His Majesty's visit would also include some of his closest friends and advisers. The king would inquire as to the sex and health of the infant and then he would perhaps declare the child's name and title(s). After the king left the confinement room he would announce the birth with details of the baby's gender. Next to be admitted were the queen's closest female relatives and the highest-ranking noble women who, after formally curtsying to the queen, showered their praises on the new royal infant. Then the king's Privy Council members, who remained just outside of the chamber, offered their congratulations and well wishes to the queen.

Announcements of the royal birth were made by the court's royal heralds; if the child was a boy, bells rang, cannons fired, and bonfires were lit. For a baby girl, the celebrations were more subdued but still festive. Messengers were sent to foreign rulers, noble families and court ambassadors would get busy writing down the details of the birth for their masters. A little princeling would also merit jousts in his honour.

Senior courtiers and Privy Council members would swear an oath of fealty to the newborn prince or princess in the presence of the king. Later, a formal swearing-in ceremony for nobility and courtiers would take place when a binding oath was made before the Archbishop of Canterbury and the king.[28]

The queen would remain in her confinement chamber for another thirty to forty days, receiving female visitors and perhaps listening to musicians play in an adjacent room. Male courtiers could not visit within the actual confinement chamber but could pay their respects from outside the room or by sending gifts to the queen. Midwives would make regular visits to the queen in the first week or two of her lying-in period to make sure all was well and to answer any questions. The royal wet nurse would have a place in the royal confinement rooms as would the infant's rockers – female servants whose sole purpose was to rock the royal cradle.

The baptism ceremony would be next on the agenda. Held within days it was a sprinkling of water or even a complete submersion and a recitation of words to erase original sin. With infant deaths a common occurrence, no parent risked delay. Godparents, often three (two of the child's sex, one of the opposite), were chosen for their spiritual clout and social ties. Royal baptism ceremonies were elaborate celebrations requiring expensive decorations for the church with orchestrated processions to the baptismal font. After the conclusion of the ceremony the guests would be escorted to the lying-in chamber where the new mother would hear words of praise for her newly baptized infant. A luxurious banquet would round out the day's festivities.[29]

The christening of Prince Edward Tudor, the son of Henry VIII and Jane Seymour, is described as taking place on 15 October, 1537, three days after his birth. He was carried to the royal chapel of Hampton Court Palace by Marchioness Lady Exeter. His half-sister, Lady Mary, was appointed as the infant's godmother. Mary was dressed in a costly cloth of silver gown, richly embroidered. The tiny prince was dressed in an elaborate gown that had a train so long it was carried by Lord William Howard and the Earl of Arundel. At least 300 nobles, foreign envoys and clerics were witness to the ceremony. The procession began with gentlemen walking in pairs carrying unlit torches followed by the children and ministers of the king's chapel. Then came knights, chaplains and members of the peerage all walking in pairs. Last came Prince Edward in the arms of Lady Exeter beneath a canopy held up by Thomas Seymour and other gentlemen of privilege. The royal child had three godfathers, Charles Brandon, Duke of Suffolk, Thomas Howard, Duke of Norfolk and Archbishop Thomas Cramner. The christening was conducted by Archbishop Cranmer and at the naming of the prince, the torches were lit and the heralds cried out, 'Edward son and heir to the King of England, Duke of Cornwall and Earl of Chester'.[30]

The procession then marched to the queen's chambers and the baby was placed in his mother's arms. Although weak from her long and arduous labour, Jane joyfully received her son, holding him a while before the king and Jane gave the infant their blessings before he was removed to his nursery.

A Tudor queen remained sequestered in her chambers for another forty days after the birth. During this interval the queen would be entertained by her kinswomen, female courtiers and by musicians playing in a nearby room. Dainty refreshments were served and the women enjoyed themselves.

The end of confinement was celebrated by the churching ceremony. Essentially the ceremony was a rite of purification and reintroduction into society for the new mother. The queen would enter the chapel veiled and a priest would sprinkle holy water over her while reciting, 'Benedicto mulieris post-partum ante ostium ecclesie'. Then the priest would recite

Psalms and speak of God's deliverance of the queen from the dangers of childbirth. This postpartum ritual had special significance for women in the sixteenth century. The queen would be accompanied by at least two other married women to the altar, then after the conclusion of the churching, a party would follow. This was a festive time of celebration for women and by all accounts a merry one.[31]

The churching ceremony has an interesting history – even a controversial one with its Jewish origins. The ritual of the churching ceremony became contentious during the Protestant era. In 1552, Hugh Latimer preached in church before the Duchess of Suffolk, 'The law [of purification] was a law made unto the Jews and not unto us; .. women in childbed be not unclean before God; neither is purification used to that end, that it should cleanse from sin; but rather a civil and politic law, made for natural honesty's sake'. In 1570, the 'Admonition controversy' raised objections due to 'Jewish remnants' in the act of churching after childbirth because 'churching of women smelleth of Jewish purification'[32]

Jewish women in both modern and ancient history all undergo a ritual immersion into a bath of natural water or specially collected rainwater after forty days postpartum. After full immersion the woman arises and recites a prayer. She is considered purified and can resume normal activities including marital relations. The next day the purified woman goes to her synagogue and recites a special prayer of thanksgiving for surviving a dangerous time in front of a rabbi and a quorum of at least ten men, though she herself remains behind a partition for modesty.

During the First (1000–586 BCE) and Second Temple eras (539 BCE –136 AD), women brought an offering of a dove sacrifice to the Temple as a means of giving thanks for surviving childbirth. Thomas Cartwright considered the churching ritual 'most Jewish and carrieth with it a strong scent of suspicion of a sacrifice'. The rite remained a popular custom among the average woman as a female bonding ritual and very few were discouraged by the churchmen who found it distasteful due to its possible origins in the Jewish religion.[33]

To summarise, the ritual of churching was an important female bonding ritual for women of the Tudor court and during the Catholic era it was condoned by the Church. Later when England began to transition to a more Protestant society the ritual was deemed unseemly because of its origins in the Jewish religion.

Chapter 3

The Queen of Hearts: Elizabeth of York

'Push, your Grace, push', the midwife urges the young woman. With a burst of strength and tremendous effort, she squeezes her eyes shut and brings into the world a perfect baby boy. "Tis a bonny boy!' the midwife declares as she cuts the navel cord and passes up the child to his mother. Elizabeth of York smiles down at her son before looking up at her own mother who has come to kneel beside the birthing stool to gaze upon her first grandchild.

'You did it, my darling. You have secured the next Tudor heir!' The two women gaze down at the little boy with the big destiny.

It would be unfair to discuss the matriarchs of the Tudor dynasty without beginning with Elizabeth of York; the beautiful mother of Henry VIII and an extraordinary queen on whose body the Tudors were conceived.

Elizabeth of York was born on February 11, 1466, at the Palace of Westminster, the eldest child of King Edward IV and Elizabeth Woodville. Astonishingly, we know the name of the midwife who delivered her: Margery Cobbe.[34] Her birth occurred during a relatively stable moment in her father's reign, following his victory over the Lancastrians at the Battle of Towton in 1461, which had secured the Yorkist claim to the throne. Edward IV, a tall and notoriously handsome monarch, had solidified his rule, but his marriage to the lovely Elizabeth Woodville, a commoner from a minor gentry family, created much controversy amongst the nobility. The Woodvilles' swift rise to prominence created derision at court, particularly with prominent men like Richard Neville, Earl of Warwick, also known as the 'Kingmaker'.[35]

As a royal princess, Elizabeth's early years were privileged, in spite of the undercurrents of political instability. As was fitting for a princess, she received her baptism at Westminster Abbey, with one of her godparents being her grandmother, Cecily Neville, Duchess of York. The court of Edward IV was young and vibrant, filled with royal pageantry as well as art and culture. Elizabeth received an excellent education, including training in music, embroidery, and religious devotion, though specific details of her childhood curriculum are scarce. Her mother, Elizabeth Woodville, the intelligent and ambitious Lancastrian queen, shaped young princess Elizabeth's understanding of courtly life and politics.

By 1470, Elizabeth's idyllic early childhood was pulled apart by the rekindling of the Wars of the Roses. The Earl of Warwick was highly disillusioned with Edward IV's management of his kingdom and his favouritism toward the Woodvilles who were allied with the exiled Lancastrian queen, Margaret of Anjou. It was her ambitious desire to restore Henry VI to the throne. In October 1470, Edward IV was forced to flee to the Low Countries, and Elizabeth Woodville, pregnant again, sought sanctuary in Westminster Abbey with her young daughters, including 4-year-old Elizabeth. This period of exile was young Elizabeth's first direct experience of the fragility of royal power. In the sanctuary, her mother gave birth to Edward, Prince of Wales (later Edward V), under precarious circumstances, and for Elizabeth, this would teach her of the vulnerabilities of women, especially royal ones, during times of crisis.[36]

Edward IV's victories at Barnet and Tewkesbury in 1471 restored the Yorkist dynasty and stability to Elizabeth's childhood. The Lancastrians' defeat and the deaths of Henry VI's heir and Henry VI himself solidified Edward IV's claim to the throne. Elizabeth was now the eldest daughter of a reigning king, and a valuable asset in the European marriage market. Her father wasted no time in entering into negotiations in order to secure the most advantageous alliances. At the tender age of 9, Elizabeth was betrothed to the Dauphin of France and was styled 'My Lady the Dauphine'.

Growing up in the opulent Yorkist court, Elizabeth was surrounded by her siblings – by 1483, her parents had produced ten children, seven of whom survived infancy, including three brothers (Edward, Richard, and

George) and four younger sisters (Cecily, Margaret, Bridget and Anne). The court was a busy hub of cultural and political activity, with Queen Elizabeth Woodville at the centre of it all. Elizabeth likely developed a close bond with her mother whose skill in navigating court intrigues would later influence Elizabeth's own approach to queenship.

The Yorkist court was not without its tensions due to the Woodvilles' influence which alienated key nobles. Edward IV's reliance on his wife's family created factions that would later destabilise the dynasty. Elizabeth, as a young princess, would have observed these dynamics, learning the art of courtly survival.

On April 9, 1483, the sudden death of her father Edward IV at the age of 40, plunged Elizabeth's life into chaos. At 17 she was no longer the daughter of a reigning king but the sister of the new monarch, her 12-year-old brother, Edward V. The transition of power should have been straightforward, but Edward IV's untimely death left the kingdom chaotic and vulnerable. The young king was under the guardianship of his uncle, Richard, Duke of Gloucester (later Richard III), who was appointed Lord Protector. Tensions between Richard and the Woodvilles escalated rapidly, as young Edward's family struggled to maintain their influence over the young king.

Elizabeth Woodville greatly mistrusted Richard's intentions. His ambitions felt threatening to the dowager queen, so again she sought sanctuary in Westminster Abbey with her children, including Elizabeth. This decision was borne out of fear. Richard indeed proved her suspicions were correct when he swiftly moved to consolidate power. In June 1483, Richard arrested and brutally executed young Elizabeth's uncle, Anthony Woodville, Earl Rivers, and her half-brother, Richard Grey. The most devastating blow came when Richard declared Edward IV's marriage to Elizabeth Woodville invalid, citing a supposed pre-contract with another woman, Eleanor Butler. This relegated Elizabeth and her siblings to the demoted status of bastards and thus ineligible to rule England. After placing his nephew, the young Richard, Duke of York, in the Tower, Richard declared himself king – Richard III – on June 25, 1483. This decree ushered in a new and humiliating status for Elizabeth, relegating her and her siblings to the margins of political relevancy. Elizabeth's brothers, King Edward V and Richard, Duke of York – known as the Princes in the Tower – were prisoned in the Tower of London, their unknown fate becoming one of history's most compelling mysteries.

By late 1483, the princes had disappeared from public view, leading his family and the public at large to presume them dead, though no actual evidence confirms their fate. For Elizabeth, the loss of her brothers was a devastating tragedy as well as a political crisis, since it undermined the Yorkist claim to the throne and left her as the most prominent surviving heir of Edward IV.

In sanctuary at Westminster Abbey, Elizabeth and her mother faced an uncertain future. The abbey's austere conditions, though safer than the outside world, were in stark contrast to the opulence and comforts of their former life at court. Elizabeth Woodville's decision to remain in sanctuary demonstrates her acute awareness of the dangers posed by Richard III's ill-gotten regime. This situation acutely harmed her daughters, who could be used as pawns in marriage alliances to give Richard's monarchy the patina of authenticity. For Elizabeth of York, this period was uncertain as well as humiliating. She was now the eldest daughter of a deposed dynasty. Her education and upbringing, however, would have created a woman of resilience and fortitude. There could be no better training for the challenges that would be lying ahead of Elizabeth after her marriage to Henry VII.

In 1484, Elizabeth Woodville and her daughters emerged from sanctuary after negotiations with Richard III. The exact terms of their release are unclear, but Richard swore an oath to protect the Woodville women. Richard promised not to imprison them again and he vowed to arrange suitable marriages for his nieces. In return, Elizabeth Woodville agreed to leave sanctuary, in essence, acknowledging Richard's kingship. For Elizabeth of York, now 18, this marked a return to comfy court life, unfortunately under her uncle's reign and not her brother's. The Yorkist court under Richard III was quite different from her father's; it was factionalised and viewed by many through eyes narrowed in suspicion.

Elizabeth's status during this period was ambiguous to say the least. She was no longer a princess in title, though she was none the less an asset with her Yorkist breeding. Rumours began circulating about Richard's intentions toward the beautiful girl, particularly after the death of his wife, Anne Neville, in March 1485. The contemporary view was that Richard considered marrying Elizabeth to secure his claim to the throne and remove her as a rallying point for Yorkist supporters. Even in 1485 this would have been scandalous, given their close kinship. Marrying his brother's daughter, whose supposed illegitimacy marked her as a bastard would have been a bizarre action on Richard's part. There are historians who believe that these rumours were simply Lancastrian propaganda to discredit Richard. But the rumours do serve to reflect the precarious position Elizabeth occupied at court. Elizabeth's own feelings on the subject are not recorded, though as a young woman raised to understand dynastic politics, she conceivably understood the potential danger and opportunity her position entailed.

During this time, Elizabeth's mother, Elizabeth Woodville had secret communications with Lancastrian exiles, particularly Margaret Beaufort, the mother of Henry Tudor, the Lancastrian challenger. These negotiations set the stage for a potential alliance between the Yorkist and Lancastrian sides, with Elizabeth of York as the pretty linchpin. Henry Tudor emerged from his exile in Brittany to usurp Richard III, a deal sweetened with the promise to marry the beautiful 18-year-old Elizabeth and unite the warring houses. This plan, probably cooked up by the mothers Elizabeth Woodville and Margaret Beaufort, positioned Elizabeth as the lovely white rose of Yorkist legitimacy, essential to Henry's claim to the throne of England. Elizabeth would have understood that it was her destiny to restore her family's honour and their path back to the throne of England.

The turning point in Elizabeth's life came with Henry Tudor's invasion in August 1485. Landing at Milford Haven in Wales, Henry rallied support from disgruntled Yorkists and Lancastrians, capitalising on their discontent with Richard III's rule. Elizabeth, though not directly involved and possibly still at Richard's court, remained an important symbol for supporters. Henry's public promise to marry her positioned his campaign as both a restoration of rightful Yorkist rule and an advancement of his own claim. The decisive Battle of Bosworth on August 22, 1485, ended in Richard III's defeat and death, paving the way for Henry to claim the throne as Henry VII.

After Bosworth, Elizabeth's status changed dramatically. Henry VII, cautious and pragmatic, delayed their marriage until January 1486. Elizabeth was by then 19 years of age; she spent the months following Bosworth in the care of her mother or at a safe location, such as Coldharbour House in London, awaiting Henry's arrangements. Her reunion with her mother, Elizabeth Woodville, would have been a moment of relief, though tempered by the lingering grief over her brothers' fate.

At the time of her marriage on 18 January 1486, Elizabeth was a figure of immense symbolic importance. Her union with Henry VII, celebrated at Westminster, was a public affirmation of the Tudor dynasty's legitimacy, blending Yorkist and Lancastrian claims. Elizabeth's obstetrical history was central to her role as a Tudor mother, beginning with the birth of her first child, Arthur, in September 1486. Her pre-marriage years laid the foundation for her strength and grace as queen consort. The challenges of her youth, from sanctuary to the intrigues of Richard III's court, forged a woman capable of managing the complexities of a new dynasty.

The imminent birth of Elizabeth and Henry's baby gave Margaret Beaufort her first opportunity to put into place her new Royal Confinement Ordinances. From the moment of quickening Margaret had been hard at work putting together the new court protocols for the lying-in. Elizabeth was the first queen to benefit from Margaret's thoughtful approach to the expectant mothers every need. Elizabeth made a formal withdrawal along with selected ladies of her court as she was showered with blessings from her priest and courtiers. Once again, Margery Cobbe appears in the records as being the attending midwife to young Elizabeth, delivering the next generation of York royalty. On the morning of 20 September, baby Arthur Tudor made his appearance.[37] Elizabeth would go on to birth six more children and enjoyed the same seemingly effortless fertility that her own mother had. There are no known stillbirths or miscarriages experienced by Elizabeth of York, although some biographers theorise that she may have had one or two miscarriages in the late 1400s or early 1500s, but no records confirm this. Elizabeth would have had a perfect record of fertility had she not died of puerperal fever a few days after giving birth to her last child in February 1503. Tragically, her death came only ten months after the death of her firstborn son, Arthur Tudor. In only seven short years, Henry VIII would become king of England and turn the well-ordered kingdom of his parents' upside down.[38]

Chapter 4

Katherine of Aragon, Wife of Sir Loyal Heart

Within the dimly lit birthing chamber, Queen Katherine struggles to sit upright, desperate for a look at her new baby. Her friend Maria de Salinas soothes her in their native language of Spanish. 'Why don't I hear my baby crying?' Katherine asks her friend. Maria does not address the question, rather she speaks gently to the young queen, reminding her to allow the midwives to complete their duties.

'Soon you shall meet your son, the midwives are cleaning him for your Grace.' Katherine knows with every bone in her body that something is wrong, terribly and irrevocably wrong. 'My baby! Bring me my baby!' she cries. 'I must see my son!' The midwife hurries back to the queen and says in a calm and quietly respectful voice, 'Your Majesty gave birth to a stillborn girl. I am sorry, your Grace.' Katherine's anguished wail fills the chamber with its heartbreaking sound. The midwife pats the queen's forehead and cheeks with a linen cloth wrung out in rosewater. She has seen many women lose their infants in her three decades of service to birthing women, but this time was different. This time the mother had failed her husband, her King and her nation.

Katherine of Aragon was Henry VIII's first queen consort. They married when she was 23 and Henry 17. This queen's reproductive history has the most information to be gleaned about the fertility problems surrounding the Tudors due to the fact that this marriage was the longest. Katherine of Aragon was the sixth child of Queen Isabella of Spain and King

Ferdinand of Aragon. Isabella and Ferdinand had long hoped to join their royal house to England as part of a diplomatic strategy that would align these great European monarchies against France. The betrothal between Arthur Tudor and Katherine was formalised in 1489 when Arthur was 3 years old and Katherine just one year older. Both Katherine and Arthur Tudor were great-great grandchildren of John of Gaunt, Edward III's third surviving son. This is understood to mean that their union would have to be granted a papal dispensation on the grounds of consanguinity. Inbreeding was prevalent amongst the nobility so dispensations from Il Papa were extremely common.[39]

Henry VII and his wife Elizabeth were overjoyed at the prospect of a Spanish Infanta as a daughter-in-law; this gave their nascent dynasty the status that it was lacking. Katherine brought a sizable dowry with her too, which pleased her in-laws greatly. An alignment with Spain helped Henry's influence in Europe; Spain was a powerful military and diplomatic European force. Queen Isabella did have a few prerequisites, however – no other claimants to the English throne would be tolerated. Edward Plantagenet, Henry's Yorkist cousin who was imprisoned in the Tower since the age of 9 (immediately following Henry's ascension to the throne) would have to be executed as well as Perkin Warbeck. Warbeck had claimed to be Richard, Duke of York, the son of Edward IV and rightful heir to the throne, as well as the brother of Elizabeth York, the king's wife. Both young men were summarily beheaded.

With Edward Plantagenet and Perkin Warbeck now out of the way, Katherine was quickly dispatched to England. Prince Arthur was said to have been thrilled with his pretty bride, as was King Henry. England rejoiced in the arrival of the Infanta, welcoming her with great fanfare as she rode into London on a snow-white mule, an animal associated with the Spanish monarchy; but given the fact that mules are sterile creatures, perhaps the choice was an unfortunate one. The people of England adored their new princess, and Katherine would remain extremely popular with her subjects for her entire lifetime.

On Sunday, 14 November 1501, Arthur married Katherine in St Paul's Cathedral. Katherine was dressed in white satin embroidered with pearls and spun gold embroidery; her long, loose auburn hair was covered with a fine white veil edged in gold and precious gems. She was escorted by Prince Henry, 10 years old at the time, to the cathedral. Arthur wore white satin to match his bride. The nuptial mass lasted for three hours.[40]

After the mass, Arthur slipped away, and Prince Henry guided Katherine outside where they were greeted by a high green mound covered in precious metals. This hill was the symbol of King Henry VII's 'rich mount' (Richmond), and Arthur stood at the top of the mound in front of a tree dressed as a king in shining armour. He was flanked by actors dressed as the king of Spain on one side and the king of France on the other, each with a tree directly behind them. From the core of the mountain a 'spring' of wine flowed downhill for the guests to partake of. The wedding party then proceeded to Baynard's Castle where there were a grand feast and a formal bedding ceremony.[41]

In the morning, Arthur joked to his companions that he was thirsty after having been 'in the midst of Spain'. There is plenty of opinions about whether or not this marriage was ever actually consummated, with Katherine herself swearing in court decades later during the Blackfriars trial in June 1529 that she was a virgin at the time of her second marriage to Henry VIII. It is unlikely in the extreme that Katherine and Arthur actually consummated their marriage for one compelling reason – Katherine was so fertile that she conceived almost immediately following her marriage to Henry VIII, and she was married nearly six months to Arthur. She swore she had not had conjugal relations with Arthur, and the lack of any pregnancy is, in my opinion, confirmation of this vow.

Sadly, Prince Arthur passed away on April 2, 1502, and Katherine became a widow at the age of 16. Why did the young Prince die? The records suggest that Arthur was not a healthy boy, and that he had an underlying medical condition. The records state that Arthur had 'a pitiful disease and sickness of deadly corruption that did utterly vanquish and overcome the blood'.[42]

Many historians suggest it was the dreaded 'sweating sickness' but this seems unlikely because that disease killed swiftly and in Prince Arthur's case, it took him nearly an entire week to succumb. Readers will see a similar pattern arise with other noble young men of this lineage, which will be thoroughly investigated in a subsequent chapter.

The next several years would be difficult for Katherine because her parents wished for her to remain in England and marry Prince Henry. The English king was less enthusiastic about this plan and told Isabella and Ferdinand that they must first turn over the entirety of Katherine's dowry before he would consider the request. The Spanish monarchs refused Henry VII's demand and poor Katherine became a pawn in this royal chess match and suffered greatly. Her mother passed away in 1504 and her father, King Ferdinand, was unsympathetic to his daughter's plight. Katherine remained in this unfortunate situation until King Henry VII's death in 1509. Then, like a hero from a fairytale, 17-year-old Henry, now Henry VIII, swooped in to save the princess by marrying her and crowning her his queen.

Katherine conceived almost immediately and the whole kingdom rejoiced at this happy news. Unfortunately, Katherine went into labour prematurely and delivered a seven-month-old stillborn girl on January 31, 1510. To add insult to injury, Katherine's physician insisted that she was pregnant with a surviving twin, so Katherine went back into her confinement chamber and stayed there until her uterine swelling went down. I wonder why an experienced midwife was not on hand to explain that the uterus remains enlarged for several weeks after birth, and Katherine was normal in this respect.

Eventually, her physician had to declare that she was no longer with child and Katherine was allowed to resume her normal life. The whole ordeal was very embarrassing for Katherine and difficult for her to explain. She wrote to her father that she had given birth to a stillborn girl and begged him not to be angry with her.[43]

This scenario demonstrates how women were blamed for their inability to birth a live child. A common myth at this time was that a stillbirth was a sign of God's displeasure, presumably with the mother. It was a difficult stigma, despite its common occurrence in a time when pregnancy was not well understood and modern prenatal care was an unknown entity. Katherine would probably learn very quickly to keep her fertility status close to her chest; it would be a good guess that when she missed a period or three, she kept this knowledge a secret. It's not inconceivable that there were early miscarriages that nobody was aware of save Katherine and her midwife. Given this obstetrical history, I conclude that Katherine had more miscarriages than were revealed in the records. Only Katherine's late-stage miscarriages became public knowledge given the fact that it would be impossible for her to hide a seven-month pregnant belly. Many theories have been offered as to why she miscarried and gave birth to multiple stillbirths. Could it have been syphilis contracted from her husband? Perhaps her diet was inadequate from too much religious fasting? Maybe she had endometriosis or other gynaecological problems? It is clear from her frequent pregnancies that she was ovulating regularly; she was very fertile, and her husband was known at this point in his life to have a high sex drive. The question remains: why was she unable to carry a baby to full term? Out of numerous pregnancies, only two babies were born alive. This is highly unusual and very frustrating without details of Katherine's gynaecological history. How anguishing it must have been for the queen to lose so many children!

How was a woman to know for certain if she were pregnant in the sixteenth century? There were no tests, ultrasounds or foetal heart dopplers and one or two missed periods were not considered anything of great significance. The pregnancy was confirmed by the 'quickening', when the baby was big enough for the mother to feel the child stirring. This subtle movement occurs somewhere between 15–20 weeks of gestation and could be the halfway point of a pregnancy. Who then can say with any certainty whatsoever how many miscarriages Katherine had? One historian, in his article about the miscarriages of Katherine of Aragon and Anne Boleyn, wrote that his research had found evidence of ten miscarriages for Katherine.[44]

A healthy baby boy was born to Henry and Katherine on New Year's Day 1511. The child was christened Henry, and survived only for a few weeks, dying on 22 February. No cause for the death was noted in the records. Infant mortality at that time was twenty to thirty percent before the age of one year.[45]

On January 31, 1511, Katherine delivered a stillborn daughter. Then in 1513, Katherine went into confinement and had another son who died shortly after birth on the seventeenth of September. The records show another pregnancy in the summer of 1514. Badoer, the Venetian ambassador, wrote to his senate in November 1514 that 'The Queen has delivered of a stillborn male child of eight months to the very great grief of the whole court'.[46]

The court must have been holding their collective breath, hoping that the queen would fall pregnant soon and give birth to a healthy, thriving infant. Cardinal Wolsey wrote to Richard Fox, Bishop of Winchester in September 1511 that 'The Queen is with child' and there is no record of confinement so the queen must have had another miscarriage. (Sir John Dewhurst). No other pregnancies were mentioned until the successful pregnancy and birth of Princess Mary on February 18, 1516. The little girl was baptised three days later to the great rejoicing of the realm. No other pregnancies were noted for Katherine until November of 1518 when she delivered another stillborn daughter.[47]

Her cycles after this miscarriage became erratic, probably due to the onset of perimenopause in my opinion, but fertility wanes slowly and so it is probable that she may have had other miscarriages until her cycles finally came to a halt in 1525. The question looms large – why would so obviously fertile a woman only have one child? It's clear from the history of Katherine of Aragon that she did have many pregnancies. What could be the deathly culprit of so many miscarriages and stillbirths? Many historians believe that Henry VIII had syphilis and that this is the root of the problem.

What is syphilis? Syphilis is a sexually transmitted disease that causes wart-like growths on both male and female genitalia. It may cause hair loss and rashes break out on the body. Urination becomes excruciatingly painful and the glands in the neck become very swollen and tender. Dreadful looking boils erupt over the entire body that excrete stinking pus. A dormant or latent phase occurs for several months, perhaps even years before grotesque tumours break out over an affected person's body; these are called gummas. The bones begin to soften, sometimes causing the nose to cave-in. Then the brain and nervous systems begin to deteriorate. Often organ failure follows which causes many patients to die of heart attacks. In pregnancy, syphilis causes stillbirths, miscarriages, neonatal death and congenital deformities of the infant. Syphilis can cause the demise of a baby within the womb at any time of gestation. Repeated miscarriage is common if a mother is afflicted with the disease. Syphilis was emerging as a major disease in the sixteenth century. So, is this the root of Katherine's obstetrical misfortunes? Upon close examination of Katherine's history, we see that there is no recorded evidence that Katherine had any symptoms of syphilis. Did King Henry VIII have this increasingly common venereal disease as some historians speculate?

Henry VIII was described as the only child of his parents that was healthy from birth. As a young man he had a light case of smallpox and a few minor fevers. Henry was an athlete of exceptional abilities; he was an expert rider, adept at tennis and had incredible stamina. His excellent health continued until he reached his forties, at which point he had a serious jousting accident in 1536. Then the king's health took a drastic turn. He was already a large man, but his accident led him to became obese and he suffered from 'sorre leggs' which his surgeons would care for by lancing his wounds, allowing the pus to flow from the ulcerated limb. There is ample evidence that Henry became increasingly more demented in his character and behaviour. During the sixteenth century doctors treated syphilis with mercury and there is no record of Henry ever receiving such treatment, nor did he have any of the tell-tale symptoms of the disease.[48]

We mustn't forget about Mary, Henry and Katherine's only surviving daughter. Children born with congenital syphilis have bone deformities, skin rashes and die early deaths. Mary lived until the age of 42 and showed no signs of congenital syphilis.

The mystery surrounding the great king's illness remains to this day, but it was most assuredly not syphilis. What then could account for the queen's abnormal obstetrical history? Using my skills as a midwife I have a few ideas. Antiphospholipid Syndrome is an autoimmune disorder wherein the body generates antibodies that target phospholipids; these are molecules that are essential to healthy blood vessels and proper cellular function. For women who have this condition, their own body produces an attack against the pregnancy causing abnormal blood clotting. To further elaborate: tiny blood clots strangle the blood vessels which supply nutrients to the placenta. A well-functioning placenta is crucial to the proper growth and survival of the embryo. If the foetus is deprived of oxygen and nutrition, then the foetus will die within the womb. This causes miscarriage, stillbirth or a condition called eclampsia which is extremely dangerous – and in the sixteenth century a fatal condition. Katherine's gynaecological history has many similarities to APS. Often women who have this autoimmune disorder experience both early and late miscarriages. Sometimes a baby may miraculously survive the pregnancy but die suddenly after birth, Katherine had a child in 1511, the 'New Year's Prince' who inexplicably passed away after less than two months. Sometimes women with this condition are able to have one or more surviving children. APS is a strong candidate for Katherine of Aragon's erratic and often tragic pregnancies. However, there are several factors not in alignment with this theory. APS dramatically reduces the possibility of a live birth without modern-day anticoagulants. Katherine had two surviving infants, one of which grew up to become Mary I of England. In addition, usually mothers who have this autoimmune disorder have miscarriages in the first trimester, and several of Katherine's pregnancies went into the second or third trimester. There is no recorded symptoms like deep vein thrombosis, strokes or other unusual clotting events which make an APS diagnosis unlikely. Likewise, there is no eclampsia which would have probably been a life-threatening crisis for the queen.

Perhaps Katherine had so many miscarriages and stillbirths because she was malnourished or under severe stress? It is true that the queen had a difficult life and certainly faced repeated emotional hardships. She was also known to fast often, being a woman of great piety, so this caused so much stress on her body that she could not carry a baby to full term. In Catholic practice during the late Medieval/early Renaissance era, fasting only meant restricting certain foods such as meat and lard, and often many people had just one meal and a late snack. Total abstinence from food was not the practice when fasting was religiously motivated. Fish, dairy, bread, and vegetables were all allowed during fast days. For pregnant women full meals were allowed but without meat. Drinking water, ale or wine was not restricted at all during fast days. Katherine would have observed religious fast days, but this seems unlikely to have been so extremely restrictive that it caused her obstetrical problems. The royal Tudor court had abundant food with a huge variety of everything from meats, fish, fowl and produce that would have kept Queen Katherine well-nourished even if she fasted on religious days. As for stress causing her reproductive woes, this in and of itself would not be enough for repeated miscarriages and frequent stillbirths; something was medically wrong here.

Queen Katherine had an unusual obstetrical history; but was she the only wife with such a history? We will now go on to examine the next wife of King Henry VIII: Anne Boleyn.

Chapter 5

Anne Boleyn: The Woman That Reformed the Tudor Court

As the wee hours of dawn cast a rose-hued glow over the magnificent grey stone manor of Blickling Hall, a newborn girl takes her first breaths of life outside the womb. 'Well, what is it?' inquires Lady Elizabeth Boleyn.

"Tis a wench, my lady, a lovely little girl,' replies the midwife as she goes to clean and swaddle the tiny infant. The baby cries in protest, suddenly thrust from her warm, watery world into this cold and drafty place.

'My husband was hoping for a boy this time,' Says Lady Boleyn. 'And Thomas does so hate to be disappointed,' she adds in a weary voice.

'Well, he will just have to accept God's will, as do we all. I have a feeling this girl is going to grow up to be a beauty, mayhap she will make a good match and bring her parents glad tidings.' Lady Elizabeth Boleyn makes a derisive noise of disbelief before falling asleep, exhausted from her travail.

Anne Boleyn was born to Elizabeth Howard and Thomas Boleyn sometime in the first decade of the 1500s. If we were to believe that the portrait of a young, dark-haired woman wearing a 'B' gold and pearl necklace painted by Joos Van Cleves and part of the Lumley inventory of 1590 was Anne Boleyn, then she was indeed lovely, with an oval face and sleek dark hair beneath a French hood. But by all accounts, Anne was more than beautiful – she was cultured, intelligent, fluent in French thanks to a childhood spent at the French court and possessed of a rapier wit. She caught the eye of King Henry VIII sometime in 1522 or 1523 when she was a newly appointed lady-in-waiting to Queen Katherine but his affections for her remained hidden until he declared his esteem for her in 1526.[49]

Henry had begun to harbour thoughts of putting his wife Katherine away in favour of a younger and more fertile wife, and Anne Boleyn captivated the king with her flashing dark eyes, quick wit and graceful manner. Anne Boleyn was unique in a court that favoured women with fair hair and blue eyes; she outshone them all with her French charm and deep intelligence. On May 8, 1527, King Henry VIII told his chief counsellor, Cardinal Wolsey, that he had serious doubts about his marriage to Queen Katherine and soon Henry would appeal for a dispensation from the Pope to divorce his wife. The king had good reason to be optimistic, the Pope had allowed Henry's sister, Margaret, to divorce her husband in the spring of 1527. The annulment was granted to Margaret after only eighteen months, so Henry probably thought he would be free to marry Anne within a couple of years, if not sooner. Unfortunately for Henry, there was political unrest between France and Spain, with Imperial soldiers unfairly taken advantage of; they went weeks without food or payment from the Holy Roman Emperor, Charles V. The soldiers began a campaign of revenge and Pope Clement, fearing for his life, fled to safety under the roof of Castle Santangelo. The Holy Roman Emperor seized the opportunity to become Europe's most powerful player and graciously allowed the Pope to stay for as long as he wished, as his prisoner.[50]

With Europe in a state of upheaval, Henry had a much more difficult time getting through to the Pope and receiving his annulment. The Holy Roman Emperor was Queen Katherine's nephew, and he was not going to allow his aunt to be put aside. Now that the Pope was under Charles's control, Henry was never going to have his way, and this was something Henry was quite unused to. Anne, at this point, had gone to live at her family estate in Kent. At Hever Castle, Anne received many ardent letters from the king begging her to become his '*Maîtresse-en-titre*', a French title which conferred status to the king's singular and powerful mistress. It's clear from Henry's correspondences to Anne that his ardour for her was growing hotter by the day. Anne's replies sadly do not exist, so we don't really know how she felt about the king's attentions, but when she doesn't accept the title of *Maîtresse-en-titre,* a surprising thing happens. The king goes so far as to hint that he would like Anne to become his wife, making her queen of England. The Tudors put tremendous stock in whatever they perceived to be 'divine will' and Anne could very well have seen this as a piece of the puzzle when deciding how to respond to Henry.

We know from Henry's response that Anne sent him a jewel wrought in gold of a maiden, storm-tossed inside of a ship, an allusion, presumably, to her internal struggle with the affair. Henry's response to this gift is his promise to be Anne's in both heart and body as well as her 'loyal servant'. The year 1528 would become a pivotal year for the relationship between Henry and Anne as well as for the court and the kingdom. Henry's convictions that his relationship with Queen Katherine was contrary to God's would be intensified. The passage of Leviticus 20:21 stating that a marriage between a woman previously married to a man's brother would lead to a childless union was Henry's lynchpin. His advisors were quick to agree to Henry's justification for dissolving his union with the queen. Cardinal Wolsey was tasked with getting an annulment from Pope Clement VII, but this was no easy task. The Pope was still being held prisoner by Charles V, and he was unwilling to go against the emperor's wishes. Wolsey was in an unenviable position, with the Pope refusing to acquiesce on one side and Henry's insistence with his patience wearing thin on the other.

Anne's position on the matter may have been ambivalent for many months but now Henry had swayed her to his side, and she could envision herself as England's next queen consort. Perhaps her reticence and refusal to become Henry's mistress fuelled his ardour beyond the point of no return; a woman refusing to bed him was anathema to the king and he decided he absolutely would have her, at any cost. If Anne strung him along deliberately in order to reach this conclusion or if she simply felt unsure of her feelings and motivations, being a very young woman, we will never know for sure.

The annulment of his marriage to Queen Katherine became Henry's Great Matter, and the king's will would be obeyed. As for the queen, she would not agree to the annulment, she believed with all her might that no earthly power could undo her marriage to the king. She feared for Princess Mary as well; what might happen to her daughter if the wedding vows were nullified? She told her daughter to stand firm.

At court, Anne was often seen with the king, and soon the court split into factions; those who favoured Anne and those loyal to the queen. The two rivals for the king's affections had separate apartments at Greenwich Palace, with Anne's attaining quasi-queen status.

In early 1528 the Pope managed to sneak out of his captivity in disguise. Now Henry hoped he would be able to gain his divorce and marry Anne. A trial would be held to decide the status of the king's marriage to Katherine, overseen by Cardinal Campeggio, sent to England by Pope Clement. This trial took place on May 31, 1529, and Katherine of Aragon made a poignant speech beseeching the king not to cast her aside. The queen reminded the king that when they were first wed, she was a true virgin in spite of her first marriage to Prince Arthur. She also referenced their many children she had given birth to, though God decided to take them as infants.

Katherine's defiant defence of her marriage, kneeling before Henry to proclaim her virginity at the time of their union, swayed many in her favour. The trial's collapse, with the case recalled to Rome, marked a turning point. Henry's frustration boiled over, and Wolsey bore the brunt of his anger. Anne, who had long suspected Wolsey of prioritising his own interests, encouraged Henry to dismiss him. Wolsey's fall in October 1529, stripped of his titles and later charged with treason, underscored Anne's growing influence.[51]

Anne's position at court became more prominent, though controversial. She accompanied Henry on progresses, and her presence created not a small amount of resentment among Queen Katherine's allies, who dubbed her 'the King's whore'. Anne's quick wit and intellectual superiority did little to quell opposition, but they captivated Henry, who admired her tremendously. Their relationship thrived on intellectual discourse. Anne was the first person to introduce Henry to reformist texts, such as William Tyndale's *The Obedience of a Christian Man*, which argued for royal, i.e. human supremacy over that of the Church. These ideas planted seeds for a break with Rome, coinciding with Henry's desire to resolve the annulment independently.

Despite their closeness, 1529 was a difficult year that would test Anne's resolve. Henry's temper was at a boiling point as the annulment stalled, and rumours began insinuating his interest in other women. Anne's ability to keep their relationship chaste was the key to preserving her bargaining power but risked alienating Henry. The couple had fiery disagreements, perhaps fuelled by sexual frustration on Henry's part, and were noted by contemporaries like Eustace Chapuys. The Imperial ambassador reported Anne's frustration with Henry's indecision to break with Rome and Il Papa. Yet Anne's hold over Henry remained strong, fuelled by his belief that she was his path to a legitimate heir and divine favour.[52]

By 1530, Henry and Anne's relationship entered a new phase, marked by Henry's willingness at last to break from Rome. The failure of Henry's diplomatic efforts to secure the annulment from Il Papa pushed toward bolder measures. Anne, alongside Thomas Cromwell, encouraged Henry to assert his authority over the English Church. Thomas Cromwell urged Parliament to continue to pressure the Church, while Anne's support for reform and her gift to Henry of Simon Fish's book *A Supplication for the Beggars* influenced Henry's views of reformation.[53]

In 1530, Henry began to explore the idea of becoming the Head of the English Church, an entirely separate entity from Rome. The couple's shared vision of a reformed Church of England deepened their relationship, blending together their personal ambition with political necessity. Anne's role as Henry's confidante grew, though her public prominence fuelled hostility from members of the peerage, like the Duke of Suffolk.

Emotions in the Tudor court were running very high as Henry took decisive steps toward making Anne his wife. Queen Katherine was banned from court, sent far away to the Hertfordshire countryside. Meanwhile, Anne's household rivalled Katherine's in splendour, and she was ennobled, granted the title of Marquess of Pembroke in 1532. These actions signalled Henry's determination to marry Anne, now elevated to a member of the peerage. They also deepened the divisions at court, with Anne's enemies including the ambassador to Spain, Eustace Chapuys, who spread rumours of her supposed immoral behaviour, referring to her as 'the whore'. Fortunately, Anne was not without staunch allies at court; her supporters included her father, Thomas, and her brother, George Boleyn, who both worked tirelessly to secure her position, as well as her powerful uncle, the Duke of Norfolk.[54]

The relationship between Henry and Anne during this period ran hot and cold – collaborative and volatile. Their mutual objective of marriage and the birth of a male heir served as a unifying force, but the delay tested their resolve. Anne's impatience and Henry's authoritative disposition caused frequent disagreements. Their shared passion for reform and their unrequited passion for each other kept their relationship intact. Anne's impact on Henry's faith especially her support for Thomas Cranmer, established her as an important, if unofficial, contributor to the forthcoming separation from Rome.

The year 1532 marked the culmination of Henry and Anne's epic manoeuvres to secure their union. Thomas Cromwell's legislative efforts, including the Submission of the Clergy, forced the English Church to acknowledge Henry's authority. The death of William Warham, Archbishop of Canterbury, allowed Henry to appoint Cranmer, Anne's chosen chaplain, to the post. These developments smoothed the way for the annulment to be resolved domestically, effectively bypassing Rome.[55]

In the summer of 1532, Henry and Anne's relationship reached a new and exciting phase. During a diplomatic trip to Calais to meet Francis I of France, Anne finally agreed to consummate her relationship with the king, a strategic move demonstrating her confidence in Henry's decision to marry her and make her his queen. By late 1532, Anne was pregnant, a development that ended the wait and forced Henry's hand. The pregnancy, with the fervent hope that Anne carried within her womb the royal male heir, made legitimising their union an urgent necessity.[56]

Henry and Anne married in a secret ceremony on November 14, 1532, conducted by Thomas Cranmer. This was an unprecedented move since Henry's marriage with Queen Katherine still remained legally intact. Anne's pregnancy, however, upended the dynamics of their relationship, transforming her from a hotly pursued love interest to the future queen and mother of the king's son and heir. Henry's devotion to Anne deepened, but the stakes could not be higher, as the success of their union now hinged on the birth of a son. On May 16, Thomas Cromwell opened proceedings at Dunstable priory in Bedfordshire to investigate the circumstances of Henry's first marriage. Just one week later, on the morning of May 23, he pronounced that the marriage was invalid and against the law of God, making Henry's union with Queen Katherine illegitimate. Henry now decided it was high time to crown Anne as his queen.[57]

The preparations for Anne Boleyn's coronation were incredibly elaborate, reflecting the event's tremendous significance as a public declaration of her queenship. Scheduled for Whitsunday, June 1, 1533, the coronation coincided with the feast of Pentecost, a deliberate choice to create an ambiance pregnant (pun intended) with religious symbolism. The planning, overseen by Thomas Cromwell and a committee of nobles, began weeks in advance, with every possible detail attended to.

The financial cost was staggering, with estimates suggesting thousands of pounds were spent. Funds were drawn from the royal treasury and supplemented by contributions from the City of London and prominent nobles. These covered the creation of Anne's coronation wardrobe, the construction of temporary structures, decorations, and lavish feasts. The scale of expenditure was intended to rival or surpass previous coronations, demonstrating Henry's devotion to Anne's inalienable legitimacy.[58]

The coronation festivities began on Thursday, May 31, with a spectacular river procession from Greenwich Palace to the Tower of London. This water pageant was an elaborate public display of Anne's queenship, designed to impress both the nobility and the common folk lining the Thames. In the middle of the day at approximately 1:00 pm, Anne boarded a richly decorated barge at Greenwich, accompanied by a flotilla of over 200 vessels.

The most astonishing feature of the procession was the 'dragon or other terrible monster', described by chronicler Edward Hall, which spouted fire and accompanied the flotilla. This mechanical marvel, a fire-breathing effigy, was a big hit with the public, symbolising the power and superior innovation of the Tudor court. Smaller boats were filled with musicians and performers, floating along with the larger vessels, entertaining the spectators.[59]

As the flotilla passed, the riverbanks erupted in celebration. Cannon salutes were fired from ships. The procession took several hours, arriving at the Tower by late afternoon. Anne disembarked and was greeted by Henry VIII, who welcomed her with a public kiss, a gesture of kingly approval. Anne spent the night at the Tower, following tradition, as it was customary for monarchs to reside there before the coronation. On the morning of June 1, Anne embarked on a grand procession from the Tower to Westminster, a distance of about two miles. This magnificent pageant was the centrepiece of the coronation festivities, designed to showcase Anne's queenship to the widest possible audience. The procession began at 8 am, with Anne exiting the Tower dressed in her coronation robes of purple velvet, furred with ermine, and wearing a coronet of gold. The Duchess of Norfolk carried her long train. Anne was carried in a litter draped with white cloth of gold, drawn by white mules. A canopy of cloth of gold, held aloft by four knights of the Garter, sheltered her from the sun's rays. Her ladies-in-waiting, dressed in scarlet and gold, followed on horseback, their mounts caparisoned in matching colours. The procession included hundreds of participants, organised in strict hierarchical order. French ambassadors, led by Jean de Dinteville, rode at the head, followed by nobles, bishops, and the king's guard in their livery.[60]

The streets of London were packed with spectators, and the city had been transformed into a stage for pageantry, with Anne Boleyn as the star of the show. At key points along the route – Gracechurch Street, Cheapside, and Fleet Street – temporary stages showcased special performances. Children dressed as little white angels sang hymns, and the city's fountains ran with wine, a symbol of abundance. Triumphal arches, inscribed with Latin verses praising Anne's virtue, were erected at key points, and the Hanseatic merchants sponsored a display featuring a mechanical fountain and a choir of mellifluous maidens. The procession continued in a stately, if somewhat slow, fashion allowing the crowd to take in the spectacle. Anne smiled and waved to the crowd, projecting a feigned confidence, hiding her, no doubt, disappointment at the cold stares of her subjects. Instead of joy there was apparent apathy in the populace. Many of the spectators displayed thinly veiled resentment; the men did not remove their caps as Anne passed them by. Chronicler Charles Wriothesley noted that while the pageantry was magnificent, 'the people showed little love' for Anne Boleyn and resented Anne's usurpation.[61] Many of the citizens still maintained fealty to Katherine of Aragon. Nevertheless, the procession was a triumph of logistics and display, reaching Westminster Hall by noon. Three ladies were chosen to speak aloud of a 'prophesy' that Anne would bear a son who would usher in a 'golden world'. Anne was visibly pregnant at her coronation, being approximately six months gone with child.[62]

The City of London was transformed for the event, streets were swept clean, and temporary stages, fountains, and triumphal arches were erected along the processional route. The Guilds of London made their own contributions to the pageantry by funding the elaborate displays. Colourful banners, tapestries, and swathes of cloth of gold were hung from buildings, adding to the festive atmosphere. The Thames, the main artery for the coronation procession, was prepared for a grand water pageant, with barges decorated in vibrant colours and adorned with royal accoutrements and banners. Westminster Abbey, the chosen site of the coronation ceremony, was decorated with more exquisite tapestries, carpets, and gold cloth. The high altar was dressed for the occasion with royal relics, and a raised platform was specially constructed for the crowning. Westminster Hall, where the coronation banquet would take place, was similarly decorated , with long tables elaborately set for hundreds of guests. Provisions for the feast included vast quantities of rich food and copious amounts of wine, the records indicate that there were purchases of venison, swans, and exotic spices for the banquet. Henry made the unusual choice to have Anne crowned with Saint Edward's crown, previously only worn by kings, symbolising Henry's determination that Anne was his uncontested queen. Anne's pregnancy was on full display with the king's astrologers (predictably) predicting a son.[63]

After the coronation festivities were over Anne resumed a quiet life at Greenwich to prepare for the birth of her child, a mere three months hence. She formally entered confinement on 26 August after hearing Mass. In spite of all the astrological predictions, the child was a little girl, and she was named Elizabeth after her grandmothers. A magnificent baptism was held for the infant princess at Grey Friars Church on 10 September, three days after her birth. Her godfather was Archbishop Cranmer and her godmothers were the Dowager Duchess of Norfolk and Marchioness of Dorset, Margaret Wotton.[64]

Anne was churched as custom demanded forty days after the birth of her daughter. Within weeks she was pregnant, probably after only one menstrual cycle or at most two. Henry had once again chosen a very fertile wife. On 5 January, Henry wrote a letter to the new German ambassador praising his new wife and boasting of Anne's 'aptnes to procreation'. Chapuys reported the queen's pregnancy to his Spanish sovereign on 28 January. Henry himself formally declared it to Chapuys at the end of February. The preparations began for a royal nursery in April at Eltham Palace, and Henry ordered a sparkling new cradle from his goldsmith, Cornelius Hayes, with artwork to be done by Hans Holbein. The king also ordered new medals to be made depicting the queen with her initials A.R. signifying Anna Regina in honour, one supposes, of the impending birth of a royal heir. It seems that the pregnancy continued well into the summer with Chapuys reporting on 27 July that the queen would enter confinement 'eminently'.[65]

But Anne did not enter confinement and there are no records of a birth. It is as if the pregnancy was there one day and gone the next, with a frustrating dearth of details of what happened to the baby. It is highly probable that a stillbirth took place suddenly and the queen was loath to tell her husband knowing he would draw comparisons to her predecessor. Anne herself was probably distressed in the extreme with the added pressure of having to appear at court sans baby or expanded belly. The feeling of failure must have been immense for Anne.

Anne did not conceive again until 1535 when there is a mention of her having 'a goodly belly' in a letter written by Sir William Kingston to Lord Lisle. Nothing else is said anywhere of this mysterious third pregnancy.[66]

Anne is known to have conceived again in the fall of 1535 but miscarried of a 15- or 16-week gestation male foetus on 28 January. This would make four pregnancies in just two years, and of course there is the possibility that she may have had other early pregnancies that would go unnoticed if the miscarriage happened very soon after conception.

The obstetrical histories of Katherine of Aragon and Anne Boleyn, the first two wives of Henry VIII, display profoundly similar reproductive challenges that defined their roles as queens. Both women faced unrelenting pressure to produce a male heir, a demand that fundamentally shaped their identities and legacies within the Tudor court. They both experienced pregnancies characterised by repeated losses – miscarriages, stillbirths, and the 'unfortunate' births of daughters in a world that prioritised sons; ultimately raining down devastating consequences for both women.

Katherine of Aragon's obstetrical history spans nearly a decade, punctuated by a series of pregnancies that followed a trajectory of early promise giving way to tragedy. Her obstetrical record includes the birth of a surviving daughter, Princess Mary, alongside multiple losses that diminished her chances of delivering the male heir Henry expected of her.

Anne Boleyn's obstetrical history, covering a shorter period from 1533 to 1536, mirrors this same pattern. Based on historical accounts and the assumption of three miscarriages, one probable stillbirth, her record includes four pregnancies:

1. September 1533: Princess Elizabeth – Anne gave birth to a healthy daughter, Elizabeth, her only child to survive.
2. Summer 1534: Miscarriage – A pregnancy ended in a miscarriage, though details are limited.
3. 1535: Miscarriage – Another miscarriage occurred, further undermining Anne's position.
4. January 1536: Stillborn son – Anne suffered a stillbirth of a male child, at around 16 weeks gestation.[67]

Anne's four pregnancies resulted in one surviving daughter, two miscarriages, and one stillbirth. So, initial success followed by devastating losses. Like Katherine, Anne's fertility is defined by a high proportion of unsuccessful pregnancies, with only one surviving child – a girl.

The similarity in their parity histories lies in the common thread of their reproductive experiences. Both queens deliver a healthy daughter – Mary for Katherine and Elizabeth for Anne. Both queens go on to face a series of losses that eroded their ability to fulfil their primary role as royal baby makers. The predominance of miscarriages and stillbirths in their records highlights the fragility of their fertility, as each loss diminished their standing and intensified the pressure put upon them to conceive again and again. This parallel pattern shows the precariousness of their positions as queens whose primary role was securing the Tudor succession.

Frequent miscarriages and still births are a shared experience between Katherine and Anne but Katherine's pregnancies, occurring over nearly a decade, reflect a relentless cycle of conception and loss, with multiple setbacks interrupting her reproductive efforts. While the specific number of her pregnancies is not known, her obstetrical history shows a sustained period of reproductive activity marked by frequent losses. Anne's four pregnancies over three years, averaging one per year, indicate a similarly intense cycle, with three of her pregnancies ending in loss (a 70 per cent failure rate). The compressed timeframe of

Anne's reproductive challenges amplified the impact of her failures, but both queens endured a persistent pattern of hope, pregnancy, and loss.

The nature of their losses further aligns their experiences. Both queens experienced stillbirths, which were particularly devastating due to the losses of fully or partially formed foetuses, sometimes identifiable as male or female. Anne's 1536 stillbirth, a baby boy, carried immense emotional and political weight with this loss of a potential male heir. Katherine's obstetrical history includes similar losses that mirror this tragic disappointment. Miscarriages, less visible but equally devastating, were also a shared experience, with Anne's 1534 and 1535 losses paralleling the setbacks in Katherine's reproductive history. These early to mid-gestation losses, obfuscated by secrecy, compounded the queens' challenges, as they demonstrated the delicate nature of their pregnancies as well as their positions as queens as producing an heir was paramount..

The gender of the lost children, where known, adds another layer of similarity. Anne's loss of a male foetus in 1536 heightened the stakes, as male heirs were the ultimate objective. Katherine's miscarried infants similarly involved the loss of potential male heirs, which increases the perception of the queen's failure in a court fixated on male succession. The shared experience of losing children, particularly boys who were the hope of the realm, highlights the identical nature of their reproductive struggles. The emotional toll of repeated miscarriages was intense for both queens, unifying them in a shared experience of grief. Each miscarriage and stillbirth represented not only the loss of a child but also a blow to their identity as queens, whose value was tied to their fertility. The physical demands of frequent pregnancies – nausea, fatigue, and the risky nature of childbirth – further intensified their suffering, as recovery periods were often inadequate due to the relentless pressure to conceive again.

Katherine's prolonged reproductive efforts took a significant physical toll, with contemporary accounts mentioning increasing exhaustion as her pregnancies progressed. The emotional impact was equally hard, as each loss deepened her sense of failure. Her devout faith naturally led her to interpret her setbacks as divine tests. Katherine sought solace in prayer, but the cumulative grief of her losses left indelible marks on her psyche. The cycle of hope and disappointment, repeated over years, created unbearable emotional burdens which prayer could not alleviate.

Anne's obstetrical history though briefer, was no less intense. Her four pregnancies in three years placed considerable physical strain on her, particularly as she faced the pressure to produce an heir in a cynical court sceptical of her legitimacy. The emotional weight of her 1534 and 1535 miscarriages, followed by the 1536 stillbirth, was crushing. The stillborn son, described in some accounts as well-formed, represented a devastating loss, both personally and politically. Reports of Anne's distress, including her fear of Henry's waning affection, paint a picture of a woman struggling with profound anxiety and isolation. The rapid succession of her losses left little time for recovery, increasing her emotional and physical vulnerability.

The two wives' shared experience of grief was worsened by the very public nature of their roles. Both women were expected to maintain a queenly countenance for the benefit of their court despite their private grief, as displays of weakness could undermine their authority. The cycle of conception, hope, and loss made for a cruel cycle binding Katherine and Anne in their private club of royal infertility. The emotional similarities are particularly striking in how both queens internalised their losses. Katherine's faith provided some relief, yet her repeated failures fuelled a sense of personal inadequacy, even as she maintained her dignity. Anne, known for her feistiness, faced a more precarious position, with her losses amplifying her insecurity in a court that questioned her legitimacy. Both queens endured unimaginable sorrow that had to remain internal lest their king and court find them inadequate.

The social pressures of the Tudor court, rooted in patriarchal expectations, amplified the significance of their obstetrical failures. As queens, Katherine and Anne were judged primarily by their ability to produce a male heir, a demand that overshadowed their other contributions. The birth of daughters – Mary for Katherine and Elizabeth for Anne – was a qualified success, as female heirs were seen as less desirable in a society wary of female rule. The failure to deliver a surviving son placed both queens under intense scrutiny, with their losses interpreted as personal and dynastic shortcomings.

Katherine's delivery of Mary was a singular triumph, but it did nothing to alleviate the pressure for a prince. Her subsequent losses fuelled perceptions that she was an inadequate queen consort, greatly diminishing her social standing. In addition, her advancing age made the possibility for more children even less likely. Similarly, Anne's successful birth of Elizabeth was a victory, but the absence of a son left her vulnerable to criticism. Her miscarriages and stillbirths, particularly the 1536 loss of a male foetus, did not go unnoticed. Both queens faced a court that equated their worth with their ability to birth healthy male children, with each loss eroding their social capital.

The unequivocal gendered nature of these expectations is plain to see in the disproportionate blame placed solely on the queens. While Henry's role in conception was acknowledged, the responsibility for successful pregnancies fell squarely on Katherine and Anne. Miscarriages and stillbirths were attributed to their personal failings, with rumours of divine disfavour circulating in both cases. For Katherine, these hurtful rumours grew over the years, as her inability to produce a male heir became public knowledge. For Anne, the rumours were more immediate, with her losses fuelling accusations of her general unsuitability to be queen. Publicly, the opinion was that God was judging her and found her lacking. The insistence that both queens must produce a male heir, coupled with the stigma of failure, bound the queens in a common struggle against an unforgiving sexist framework.

The court's reaction to their daughters' births further illustrates this similarity. Mary and Elizabeth, though healthy and significant in their own right, were seen as insufficient in a society that prioritised male succession. The muted celebrations following their births contrasted with the intense disappointment of their subsequent losses and highlight the parallel social pressures Katherine and Anne faced. Through no fault of their own, both wives were seen as abject failures in the game of strategic reproduction.

The political consequences of their failures were devastating, as their inability to produce a male heir undermined their positions and provided pretexts for their removal. The underlying dynamic was the same: their miscarriages and stillbirths were cynically exploited within a court desperate to secure the succession.

Katherine's repeated losses eroded her standing, as the lack of a male heir gave Henry the excuse to question the validity of their marriage. Her failure to produce a surviving son was used as evidence of God's disapproval, promoting political manoeuvres to replace her. The political ramifications of her obstetrical record were significant, as her inability to fulfil the dynastic imperative reshaped the court's priorities. Years of losses led Henry to justify seeking a new queen.

Anne's parity failures had swifter and more dramatic consequences. Her 1534 and 1535 miscarriages weakened her position, but the 1536 stillbirth was a catastrophic blow. The loss of a male foetus, coinciding with Henry's growing interest in Jane Seymour, provided the impetus for her downfall. Her enemies capitalised on her reproductive failures to orchestrate her arrest and execution on fabricated charges of adultery and treason. The political narrative surrounding her losses framed her as inadequate, echoing the criticism levelled at Katherine. The speed of Anne's downfall, driven by the intensity of her obstetrical failures in a relatively short period, is different from Katherine's gradual decline, but the root cause was the same: the absence of a male heir.

In both cases, the failure to produce a surviving son transformed these women's personal tragedies into political liabilities. The queens endured constant insecurity in their roles due to their reproductive failures being used against them by a dynasty-focused king and court. For Katherine, her losses provided a theological and political rationale for her displacement, while for Anne, they served as a pretext for her elimination. The parallel political consequences of their obstetrical histories highlight the extent to which their worth was tied to their fertility, with devastating outcomes for both queens.

Chapter 6

Jane Seymour: The Queen Who Gave the King a Prince

I did it! I am exhausted but euphoric when the midwife hands me my little boy, freshly washed and swaddled, dressed in the lawn gown and cap that I lovingly embroidered for him these past months. I look down into my baby's blue gaze and I can see he recognizes his mother.

'Hello my love, hello! How long I have waited to meet you, my familiar stranger!' I coo to him, breathing in the top of his pretty, wispy blonde head – he smells sweet and new and fresh. The most heavenly scent in the world I think to myself. How proud his papa will be! He will surely crown me queen now.

Jane Seymour was born around 1508, although her exact birth date was not recorded. We have educated estimates ranging from 1504 to 1509; the most commonly accepted years are 1508 or 1509, based on contemporary accounts and her age at marriage. She was born at Wulfhall, the Seymour family estate in Wiltshire, though some sources suggest West Bower Manor in Somerset as a possibility. Her father, Sir John Seymour, was a knight and a respected member of the gentry, well known and highly respected for his military service under Henry VII and Henry VIII. Her mother, Margery Wentworth, descended from a noble lineage, including a connection to King Edward III through her maternal grandfather, making Jane a fifth cousin to Henry VIII. The Seymour family was not among the highest nobility, but they were ambitious and well-connected, owning numerous manors and maintaining a presence at court.[68]

Jane was one of ten children, six of whom survived to adulthood- an amazing achievement in an era of high infant mortality. Her surviving siblings included Edward Seymour, who later became Duke of Somerset and Lord Protector, and Thomas Seymour, who rose to Lord Admiral and married Henry VIII's sixth wife, Catherine Parr. Growing up at Wulfhall, Jane's education was typical of a woman of her time. Unlike Henry's first two wives, Katherine of Aragon and Anne Boleyn, who were highly educated, Jane's literacy was limited; she could read and write her name but she was not fluent in any other language but English. Her training focused on skills deemed essential for women: needlework, household management, and religion. Her needlework, in particular, was renowned for its beauty and intricacy, with some pieces surviving until 1652, when they were recorded as being given to Seymour relatives.

Jane was raised in a traditionally Catholic family who upheld traditional values, which significantly influenced her conduct and character during her later years at court. Her mother's royal ancestry and her father's proximity to the king as his body servant and gentleman of the bedchamber granted the family with access to the king's ear, allowing them to find coveted positions at court. Jane's upbringing prepared her to serve the queen at court and to secure an advantageous marriage, raising her family's status.[69]

Jane Seymour's journey to the royal court began around 1527 or 1529, when she became a lady-in-waiting to Queen Katherine of Aragon, Henry VIII's first wife. This role placed her in the queen's household, where she attended to Katherine's needs, participated in court entertainments, and unobtrusively watch the political and religious upheavals of the time. The early 1530s were turbulent, as Henry sought to annul his marriage to Katherine to wed Anne Boleyn, a decision that led to England's break with the Catholic Church. Jane was raised as a devout Catholic girl, and must have sympathised with Katherine's plight, though nothing exists in the records of her words or deeds exemplifying this opinion.

By 1532, Anne Boleyn became queen, and Jane transitioned to serve in her household. This shift put her at the heart of a more glamorous and fashionable court, different from Katherine's more sober entourage. As a lady-in-waiting to Anne, Jane witnessed the volatile relationship between Henry and his second wife, whose sharp wit and assertiveness contrasted with Queen Katherine's wifely subservience. Contemporary accounts describe Jane as pale and plain, with one observer noting she was 'no great beauty', yet her gentle and obedient nature began to draw the king's attention. Her time serving both queens gave her unique insight into the dangers and opportunities of court life, as well as Henry's growing desperation for a male heir.

Henry VIII's interest in Jane Seymour emerged in 1535, perhaps during a royal visit to Wulfhall in September of that year. By this time, Anne Boleyn's position was precarious; she had failed to produce a surviving male heir, and she had had her third miscarriage in January 1536, a tragedy with the most dire consequences for Anne. Jane, with her modest demeanour and fertile family background – her mother had borne six sons – presented an appealing contrast to Anne's fiery and independent temperament. Historians debate whether Jane actively sought the king's favour or was a pawn of her ambitious family, particularly her brothers Edward and Thomas, who may have viewed her as a means to elevate the Seymours' status.[70] Jane's refusal to become Henry's mistress, a stance she maintained when he sent her a letter and a purse of gold, impressed the king. She declared her honour was her greatest treasure, a move taken right out of Anne Boleyn's book of How to Entice a Monarch. This curated display of maidenly virtue, whether genuine or calculated, fired up Henry's attraction. By early 1536, as Anne was facing accusations of adultery and treason, Jane was moved into royal apartments, a clear sign of Henry's intentions. On May 19, 1536, the day of Anne Boleyn's execution, Henry and Jane were secretly betrothed at Hampton Court Palace. Eleven days later, on May 30, 1536, they married privately at the Palace of Whitehall in London.

The unseemly speed of the marriage created much court gossip, with some believing Henry had orchestrated Anne's downfall to wed Jane. Or, maybe like Anne, Jane was already pregnant with the king's child, necessitating a swift marriage. While no definitive evidence supports Jane's direct involvement in Anne's demise, her family's strategic positioning and Henry's actions suggest a coordinated effort to replace Anne with a more compliant and hopefully more fertile queen. Jane's marriage brought the Seymours closer to the throne and paved the way for her short but impactful reign.

Jane Seymour's tenure as queen consort, from May 30, 1536, to October 24, 1537, lasted just seventeen months. Unlike her predecessors, she was never crowned, possibly due to financial constraints or Henry's caution after Anne's fall. Her motto, 'Bound to Obey and Serve', demonstrated her submissiveness; she presented herself as a dutiful and subservient wife, avoiding the political shenanigans that had doomed Anne.[71] Jane implemented stringent behavioural standards at court, prohibiting the elaborate French fashions preferred by Anne and instituting regulations regarding her women's dress, right down to the permitted number of pearls on their skirts. Her household was characterised by religious observance and modesty, aligning with her traditional convictions.

Jane preferred her family over courtiers, as shown by her closest bonds being with her sister, Elizabeth Seymour, and her sister-in-law, Anne Stanhope. Her limited education and lack of political ambition distinguished her from Anne, who had engaged in diplomacy and relished religious debates. However, Jane was not entirely passive. In October 1536, during the Pilgrimage of Grace – a northern uprising against Henry's religious reforms – she reportedly pleaded for the restoration of monasteries, a bold move that revealed her Catholic sympathies. Henry rebuked her sharply, warning her to avoid the fate of her predecessors, and Jane meekly retreated from further interference. Her most significant contribution as queen was her effort to reconcile Henry with his eldest daughter, Mary, who had been declared illegitimate after Katherine's annulment.[72] Jane's mediation was responsible for returning Mary to her father's favour, but not to the succession. This was Jane's diplomatic skills at work; something she felt was appropriate given her overt subservience to her husband.[73]

Jane's primary duty as queen was to provide Henry with a male heir, a goal that defined her marriage. Her shotgun wedding suggests the possibility of a pregnancy that, if it existed, went the way of so many other Tudor pregnancies and simply did not progress. In December 1536, she reportedly suffered a stillbirth, a setback that heightened pressure on her to conceive again. But in March 1537, a new pregnancy was announced, and Henry took great care to ensure her comfort, pampering her with delicacies like quails from Calais to satisfy her cravings. Jane's pregnancy was a source of national hope, as Henry, now in his mid-forties, fairly old by Tudor standards, had waited nearly three decades for a legitimate son.

On October 12, 1537, after a gruelling labour lasting two days and three nights, Jane gave birth to a healthy boy at Hampton Court Palace.

The child, named Edward after St Edward the Confessor, was christened on October 15 in a lavish ceremony attended by his half-sisters, Mary and Elizabeth. Jane, though weakened, participated from her bedchamber, wrapped in furs. The birth was a triumph for Jane, fulfilling Henry's greatest ambition and securing her place as queen. Celebrations swept through England, with church bells ringing and feasts held to mark the arrival of the long awaited princeling.[74]

Tragically, Jane's triumph was short-lived. Within days of Edward's christening, she fell ill. Her attendants were blamed for allowing her to catch cold or eat unsuitably rich foods. Despite efforts to save her, Jane's condition worsened, and she died on October 24, 1537, just twelve days after giving birth. She was between 27–29 years old.[75]

Henry was devastated, retreating into mourning and wearing black for three months, a rare display of grief for him. Jane's funeral, held on November 12, 1537, at St George's Chapel, Windsor Castle, was a grand affair, the only one of Henry's wives to receive a queen's burial. Mary, Jane's stepdaughter, served as chief mourner. Henry later chose to be buried beside Jane, a decision interpreted as both sentimental and political, reinforcing Edward's legitimacy as heir. Jane's death cemented her image as Henry's favourite wife, a perception bolstered by her success in producing a son and her brief tenure, which left no time for marital discord.[76]

Jane Seymour's legacy is inseparable from her son, Edward VI, who ascended the throne in 1547 at age 9. Her brothers, Edward and Thomas Seymour, used their connection to the king's heir to gain power and influence, with Edward Seymour serving as Lord Protector during Edward's minority. The Seymour family's sway helped steer England toward Protestantism, as Edward VI's reign advanced the Reformation. Jane's role in reconciling Henry with Mary also had lasting effects, reestablishing relationships within the royal family.[77]

Historically, Jane has been portrayed as both a passive figure and a subtle strategist. Early accounts praised her gentle character, while modern historians often highlight her moral courage, as seen in her plea for the Pilgrimage of Grace rebels. Jane's image as Henry's 'true love' stems from his mourning and burial choice, but this is an oversimplification of her story. Her marriage, like those of Henry's other wives, was made by political and dynastic imperatives. Her limited education and conservative demeanour made her a safe choice for a king weary of assertive queens. But it would be a mistake to underestimate her achievements such as advocating for Mary and challenging Henry on religious policy. Jane Seymour, once a simple country girl, adeptly navigated court politics with modesty and piety. Her brief reign as queen was transformative; she secured Henry VIII's favour and gave birth to his long-desired male heir.

The Birth of Edward VI

On October 9, 1537, in the dimly lit birthing chamber of Hampton Court Palace, Jane Seymour, third wife of King Henry VIII, entered labour, her cries echoing through the tapestry-draped walls as she struggled to deliver the male heir England and its king demanded. Her travails, stretching over two and a half days until Edward VI's birth at 2:00 a.m. on October 12, was a monumental test of endurance, marked by a dramatic clash between experienced midwives and the king's physician, Dr Butts, who swooped in and pushed out the queen's attendants.[78]

As twilight fell on October 9, 1537, Jane's labour began. 'The Queen's grace fell in travail' that day, a gruelling ordeal culminating in Edward's birth at 2:00 am on October 12. The labour spanned 'two days and three nights', a marathon that tested the limits of Jane's endurance.[79]

A flicker of insight comes from the Exchequer Records which document payments for 'torches and candles' on October 9, illuminating the chamber as the midwives worked through the night. The Household Accounts of Henry VIII list payments to 'four gentlewomen and others' attending Jane, this suggests a bustling chamber where midwives watched over the queen, their presence a steady anchor amid Jane's mounting pain.[80]

The midwives, whose identities are obscured in the historical records, maintained their authority in the early hours. The Household Accounts offer no names, but a letter from Sir John Russell to Cromwell, dated October 10, mentions 'Mistress Alice', paid for 'service to the Queen's grace in her travail'. Perhaps Alice is a senior midwife, her presence hints at a figure of authority. The midwives, perhaps four or five based on payment records, rotated duties, some pressing warm cloths to Jane's back, while others might have been preparing linens or herbal infusions, their efforts bolstered by years of deliveries.[81]

On October 10, Jane's labour intensified. The midwives, as inferred from their typical roles, encouraged her to squat or lean on a birthing stool, in order to ease the baby's descent. 'Diverse women' are mentioned crowding the birthing chamber. The Exchequer Records record payments for 'rushes and cloths' on October 10, hint at membrane rupture or bleeding, the midwives scrambling to keep the chamber clean. A midwives' strategy was patience, letting labour unfold naturally, but as Jane's strength waned, her desperation must have intensified.[82]

Outside the chamber, Sir William Butts, Henry VIII's trusted physician, waited, his presence a silent, oppressive presence. The Household Accounts (October 1537) confirm payment for his attendance, and a letter from Russell to Cromwell, dated September 1537, places him at Hampton Court before labour began. A privy purse expense on October 11 reveals a critical detail: an urgent payment to Butts for 'physic' during Jane's labour. This payment, obscure but telling, hints at a growing concern.[83]

A French ambassador's dispatch, Charles de Marillac to Francis I, dated October 13, gives us this insight: Jane 'suffered greatly', the labour 'longer than expected', words that capture the chamber's mounting stress. A courtier's letter from Lord Lisle to Cromwell, dated October 11 reports 'great travail continuing', the court rife with worry as Jane grew weaker.[84]

The situation undergoes a dramatic shift at this juncture, the midwives, sensing Jane's weakening resolve, possibly advised rest, prompting her to lie down to conserve energy, after they checked the baby's position. But Butts, pacing outside, grew impatient. The privy purse payment on October 11 suggests he intervened, ordering a remedy – perhaps a stimulant like ergot, known in this period to strengthen contractions, although it was risky for both mother and child. 'Messengers sent in haste' on October 11 implies urgent communication, Butts was summoning additional supplies or consulting Henry's advisors. The queen's midwives may have protested, their experience warning of overtaxing Jane, but Butts' royal mandate silenced them. This intervention, though undocumented in explicit terms, is more than plausible given the payment to Butts and Jane's protracted labour. There is mention of a shift in Jane's energy, the term used was 'much labour' before a sudden resolution, suggesting an accelerated third stage of labour. It is my educated opinion that the baby was in an occipital posterior position and the child's presentation necessitated skilled shifting of the head in order to get him out. I can see the midwives working to get the head in a more favourable position just before Butts demands to take over the birth.

The chamber, once a well-ordered room governed by the midwives' authority, became a battleground, the midwives' voices drowned out by Butts' commands. A letter from Sir William Fitzwilliam to Cromwell, dated October 12, 1537, references 'doctors attending Jane'.[85]

As midnight passed on October 11, Jane's labour reached its climax. 'The child was delivered with speed once the hour came', suggests that, after the prolonged ordeal, the final stage was rapid, possibly due to all of the midwives' hard work at turning the mal-positioned baby just before Butts' intervention.[86] Did the midwives' skills ensure the baby's safe emergence, but the accelerated pace bore the physician's imprint? It is impossible to know for certain.

At 2:00 am on October 12, Edward VI was born, his first newborn cry piercing the chamber's stuffy, stagnant air. The birth followed 'great travail'.[87] No source specifies the baby's presentation – head-first or breech – but the attendants would have cleared his airways, cut the umbilical cord, cleaned and swaddled him. A Privy Council letter, dated October 12 declares Edward 'a goodly prince' without defects, proof of the midwives' success despite the physicians' override.[88]

A later myth claims Jane underwent a caesarean section, causing her death. No original source supports this. Caesareans were fatal in 1537 and not performed on living women. Post-delivery, the midwives cleaned Jane and moved her to bed, her exhausted body limp and feeble. Jane was 'weak' but alive for Edward's christening on October 15, suggesting initial stability. Attendants monitored bleeding and offered nourishment, though a letter from Russell to Cromwell on October 24 faults attendants for unspecified errors. After the christening, visits by the nobility were concluded, Edward was handed over to nursery attendants, per court etiquette. Jane died on October 24.[89]

Jane Seymour's marathon labour, ending with Edward VI's birth on October 12, 1537, was a singular drama of endurance and conflict. The midwives, led perhaps by 'Mistress Alice', managed the early labour with skill, but on October 11, Doctor William Butts took control of the birth, his urgent medicines and commands hastening the birth at Jane's peril. Obscure records, exchequer payments, and various letters, all hint at the tension in the birthing chamber where female expertise was forced to bow to male authority.[90]

Queen Jane's mysterious death at twelve days postpartum has invited a lot of speculation, but unfortunately historians are not medically trained individuals, and every theory about how Jane died has been, in my opinion, incorrect. Original sources provide a fragmented but critical picture of Jane Seymour's postpartum condition from October 12 to October 24, 1537, documenting her initial recovery, gradual decline, and sudden collapse. Below is a comprehensive list of every symptom and observation reported by contemporaries, drawn from primary and near-contemporary records, presented chronologically to trace queen Jane's decline.

- October 12–15, 1537: **Initial Exhaustion**
- Immediately after delivering Edward VI on October 12, Jane was 'weak' but sufficiently stable to participate in his christening on October 15. The official record describes her lying in state in her chamber, wrapped in furs, and this suggests that she was conscious and able to fulfil her role, though physically drained from her 48-hour labour. No specific symptoms like fever or bleeding are mentioned, indicating no immediate life-threatening condition. A retained placenta causes haemorrhage and in the sixteenth century, sure and swift death. Postpartum uterine infection (puerperal fever) causes immediate fever, and death follows within a week though often sooner. Jane did not have a fever. Jane 'brought forth a prince' and survived the birth, with no mention of acute distress in the first postpartum days.
- October 17, 1537: **Onset of Delirium and Weakness**
- By October 17, Jane 'waxed sore sick', with symptoms like 'delirium' and increased 'weakness'. The term 'delirium' suggests mental confusion or disorientation, a significant sign potentially linked to systemic illness, dehydration, or electrolyte imbalance. The increasing weakness shows a decline from her earlier condition, pointing to a progressing illness.[91]
- October 18, 1537: **Shortness of Breath and Abdominal Pain**.
- A lesser-known letter from Lord Lisle to Thomas Cromwell, dated October 18, 1537 provides critical details of Jane's status, noting she suffered from 'shortness of breath' and 'pains in the belly'. These symptoms suggest respiratory distress, possibly secondary to systemic illness, and gastrointestinal involvement, a clue for

what will be later called her sudden 'flux'. The abdominal pain, unique to this important source, indicates early digestive distress, predating the severe diarrhoea (flux) reported later.[92]

- October 22, 1537: **Great Weakness**.
- A letter from Sir William Fitzwilliam to Cromwell, dated October 22, 1537, describes Jane as experiencing 'great weakness' and describe ongoing 'pains in the belly'. The persistence of abdominal pain, with increased weakness, indicate a worsening condition, definitely gastrointestinal. Fitzwilliam's report, written close to the event, describes the severity of Jane's illness.[93]
- October 23, 1537: **Sudden Flux (Diarrhoea)**
- The pivotal source, a letter from Sir John Russell to Thomas Cromwell, dated October 24, 1537 states that on October 23, Jane experienced 'an naturall laxe' (diarrhoea), that was initially believed to improve her condition, as it was perceived as purging 'corrupt humours'. However, 'toward night', her condition deteriorated rapidly, leading to her death. The 'laxe' or 'flux' explicitly indicates severe diarrhoea, a symptom of intestinal infection, and its sudden onset mark a critical turning point.[94]
- October 24, 1537: **Sudden Malady and Death**
- A dispatch from the French ambassador, Charles de Marillac, to Francis I, dated October 25, 1537, describes Jane's death as resulting from 'a malady that came suddenly', with courtiers noting 'neglect' in her care. While not specifying symptoms, the word 'sudden' matches up with the rapid decline following the 'flux'. There were also references to a 'disorder in the Queen's body' before her death, pointing to internal distress, no doubt the 'flux' or related gastrointestinal symptoms. The Exchequer Records note 'messengers sent in haste' on October 23, signalling a crisis, consistent with the flux's escalation.[95]

Summary of Symptoms

- Weakness: Noted immediately post-delivery (October 12) and worsening by October 17–22
- Delirium: Confusion or disorientation starting October 17
- Shortness of Breath: Respiratory distress reported October 18
- Pains in the Belly: Gastrointestinal pain from October 18–22

- Sudden Flux (Diarrhoea): Severe diarrhoea on October 23, initially seen as benign but fatal
- Disorder in the Body: Vague internal distress before death
- Sudden Collapse: Rapid deterioration on October 23–24

These symptoms – neurological, respiratory, and gastrointestinal – suggest a systemic illness. It was almost certainly an intestinal infection, progressing over days and culminating in a fatal crisis.

The Role of 'Unmeet Meats' and Jane's Weakened Condition

The 'sudden flux' and associated symptoms point to an intestinal infection, probably dysentery (caused by bacteria such as Shigella or Salmonella), with the 'unmeet meats' and Jane's weakened postpartum state allowing a dangerous pathogen to breed unchecked. The sources, combined with sixteenth-century medical context, show how these factors converged to cause her death, exacerbated by Dr Butts' 'remedies'.

'Unmeet Meats' and Pathogen Introduction

Russell's letter explicitly blames Jane's attendants for giving her 'unmeet meats' or allowing her to 'take cold', suggesting dietary mismanagement which introduced a deadly pathogen. In 1537, 'unmeet meats' referred to inappropriate or contaminated foods, such as spoiled meat, broth, or fruit, common in Tudor kitchens where sanitation was poor and nobody ever washed their hands after using the bathroom. Postpartum diets for queens were restricted to bland, easily digestible foods like caudle (a spiced gruel) or light broth, as advised in *The Byrth of Mankynde*, to avoid taxing the body.[96] However, mishandling – for example, using contaminated water or storing food improperly – could introduce bacteria like Shigella, common in crowded courts. Marillac's letter confirms this, noting 'neglect' in Jane's care, possibly linked to food preparation by the kitchen staff.[97]

The Household Accounts record payments for meals sent to Jane's chamber, including 'poultry and fruits' during confinement, which, if improperly handled, could harbour pathogens. Dysentery, a common sixteenth-century illness, spreads via contaminated food or water, causing bloody diarrhoea, abdominal pain, and fever. Jane's abdominal pain, as reported by the aforementioned Lisle and Fitzwilliam, began days before the flux, indicating an incubation period of 2–7 days, consistent with dysentery contracted via 'unmeet meats' early in her confinement, around October 10–12.[98] The crowded, poorly sanitised environment of Hampton Court, with servants mishandling food and also soiled bedding, definitely increased the risk, as *The Byrth of Mankynde* warns of 'corrupt meats' causing 'fluxes' in postpartum women.[99]

Jane's Weakened Condition

Jane's 48-hour 'difficult travail', left her physically exhausted and immunocompromised, leaving her more vulnerable to infections. Prolonged labour requires intense exertion, which depletes a woman's energy reserves and stresses the immune system. Jane's initial weakness demonstrates this. Her confinement – standard for queens – involved prolonged bed rest, limited mobility, no fresh air and zero sunlight, plus a restricted diet, all of which caused her to become weaker.

Confinement diets, which seem to be low in protein and fresh produce, could cause nutritional deficiencies, further impairing the optimal functioning of Jane's immune system. The Household Accounts list payments for 'caudles' and 'light meats', but if these were insufficient or contaminated from unwashed hands, they exacerbated Jane's frailty. Immobility during confinement, lasting from September 16 to October 24, would have slowed down her digestion and impaired her circulation, ultimately exacerbating the gastrointestinal issues. Jane's weakened condition, combined with a pathogen (in my opinion Shigella or E-coli) from 'unmeet meats', created the perfect storm for an intestinal infection to take hold, manifesting as abdominal pain by October 18 and escalating to the 'sudden flux' on October 23.[100]

Dr William Butts' treatments would have been primarily bloodletting, which only served to weaken Jane more and hasten her death. The Household Accounts confirm payments to Butts and apothecaries from October 17–24, and a privy purse expense details 'diverse medicines' supplied, indicating sixteenth century cures like bloodletting, purgatives, or cordials, standard humoral remedies for 'flux' or fever.[101] Bloodletting, used to purge 'corrupt humours', involved removing blood, reducing blood volume and exacerbating dehydration in a patient with severe diarrhoea. Purgatives, another common sixteenth-century treatment, could worsen fluid loss, as they were used to 'cleanse' the bowels, counterproductive in the extreme for dysentery. The Exchequer Records noting 'messengers sent in haste' on October 23 suggest a crisis, triggered by Dr Butts aggressive treatments following the flux. Butts, guided by humoral theory, saw the 'laxe' as a beneficial purge per Russell's letter, but his subsequent interventions accelerated Jane's collapse by worsening dehydration, leading to hypovolemic shock or sepsis.

Jane's symptoms exactly trace the arc of an intestinal infection, probably dysentery.

- October 12–15: Weakness from labour reflects physical depletion, increasing infection risk.
- October 17: Delirium and worsening weakness suggest systemic effects, perhaps early dehydration or bacterial toxins from an incubating infection.
- October 18–22: Shortness of breath and abdominal pain indicate gastrointestinal distress and hypoxia from fluid loss.
- October 23: Sudden flux marks severe diarrhoea, depleting fluids and electrolytes.
- October 24: Rapid collapse reflects hypovolemic shock or sepsis, with 'disorder in the body' as a final gastrointestinal marker.

Dysentery, contracted via 'unmeet meats', aligns with this progression, as its 2–7-day incubation matches symptoms emerging around October 17, culminating in the flux. Jane's weakened state enabled the pathogen to proliferate, and Butts' remedies, particularly bloodletting, hastened her demise by intensifying dehydration.

To ensure thoroughness, other causes of death that I considered were:

- Pulmonary Thromboembolism: A clot could cause sudden death and shortness of breath, but the 'sudden flux' and abdominal pain describe gastrointestinal distress.
- Delayed Postpartum Haemorrhage or Puerperal fever: No source reports bleeding, and Jane's ability to receive christening guests' attendance rules out acute blood loss. Additionally, there was no mention of fever or uterine pain which rules out an infection of the uterus.

- Nutritional Deficiency: Scurvy or anaemia lacks evidence- no source talks about bleeding gums or chronic lethargy, unlike Jane's flux and delirium.
- Non-Intestinal Infection: Pneumonia or other infections don't match the flux or abdominal pain.
- Cardiac Failure: No signs of chest pain or oedema, and Jane's age (approximately 27) reduces the likelihood of a heart attack.

The 'sudden flux' and gastrointestinal symptoms make dysentery by far the most compelling diagnosis.

Jane Seymour's death on October 24, 1537, was caused by an intestinal infection, probably dysentery, triggered by 'unmeet meats' and enabled by her weakened postpartum state, as demonstrated by her symptoms – weakness, delirium, shortness of breath, abdominal pain, and a 'sudden flux'. The flux, noted in Russell's letter, indicates severe diarrhoea, from a pathogen introduced via contaminated food, and accelerated by Dr Butts' bloodletting and harmful remedies, per the Household Accounts and privy purse expenses.[102] Jane's prolonged labour and long confinement left her terribly vulnerable, allowing the infection to progress to hypovolemic shock or sepsis. Obscure clues, like Fitzwilliam's 'pains in the belly' confirm this diagnosis and I am convinced that Jane Seymour died of what essentially amounts to food poisoning.

The Family Tree of the Habsburgs

(Scientific Inbreeding Pedigree of the Habsburg Dynasty)

Simple black and white line diagram showing branches and intermarriages (focusing on the Spanish line extinction).

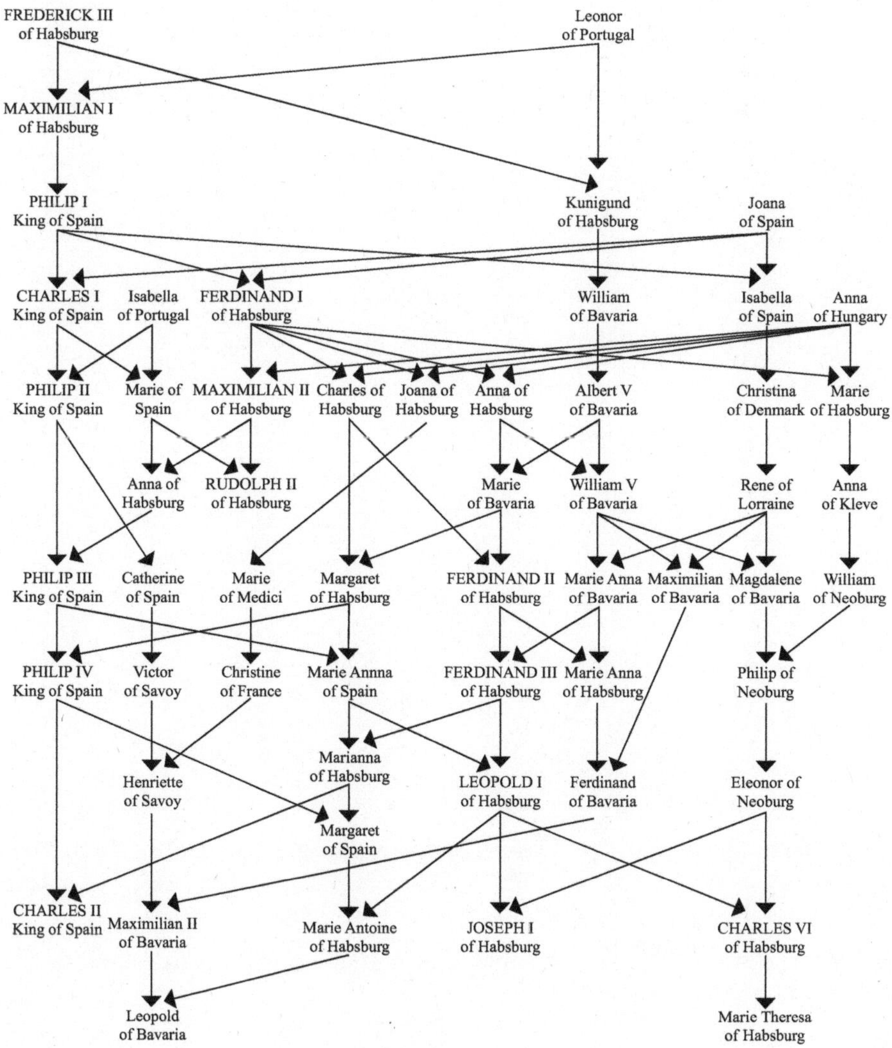

The Family Tree of the Habsburgs

[illegible]

PART 2

THE TYRANNY OF INHERITANCE

Chapter 1

Jacquetta's Curse

When the blood of a King spills red, it does not runneth pure. It bleeds secrets – silent mutations passed through the wombs of Queens until empires crack and the blood becometh dust.

As the long shadow of Elizabeth of York fades, a new inheritor rises, a golden prince whose reign began with joy and the promise of a fertile new beginning. King Henry VIII and Katherine of Aragon seemed like the perfect match; the merging of two of Europe's great monarchies as well as the wedding of two beautiful young royals. Sadly, the joy would give way to despair as Katherine suffered the loss of many infants. Henry's reign would be defined not by power or politics but by reproductive calamity. What if the cause of so much tragedy was hidden, not in scandal, but in Henry's very blood?

Modern science gives us the opportunity to revisit the Tudor cradle through a new lens – one that was not available to the midwives and physicians of the sixteenth century. The next few chapters will reexamine the marriages of Henry's first three wives as case studies in a provocative hypothesis: that Henry VIII carried a rare and deadly Kell-positive blood antigen.

If true, this simple genetic fact could explain decades of miscarriages, stillbirths and maternal suffering. It could reshapc how we understand the Tudor obsession with heirs – not as divine punishment but as the tragic consequence of one king's invisible inheritance.

Before we begin to examine the theory of blood group incompatibility, we must first understand reproductive strategy. In evolutionary biology, reproductive strategy refers to the ways in which a species or an individual within a species maximises its chance of passing on its genes to its offspring. These strategies are shaped both by biology and environment, and they influence everything from the number of offspring to the timing of reproduction to the care given to babies after birth. Reproductive strategy is complex; it can be influenced by fertility windows and maternal age, infant survival rates, access to essential resources, cultural climate and social structures. In animals, some species reproduce rapidly and often, for example rabbits, while others invest heavily in just a few offspring, like elephants and people. These are known as r-strategies and k-strategies, respectively. Human beings, especially in high status circles or societies with lots of resources, often follow a k-strategy with fewer births and higher investments per child. In early modern Europe, and particularly in royal families, something unusual occurred: women were pressured to bear as many children as possible, not to ensure genetic diversity, but to secure dynastic survival. Queens had to farm out their babies to wet nurses, while binding their own breasts to stop their own milk from flowing. Each child was a pawn in a political game, and each miscarriage was a crisis. Thus, royal reproductive strategy was biological, social, and strategic all at once. No dynasty was more shaped by reproductive failure than the Tudors. Just as the natural world is shaped by invisible genetic forces, so too were the royal houses of Europe, but where wild creatures evolved according to nature, royal women were asked to overcome nature itself.[103]

The Tudor Dynasty, reigning over England from 1485 to 1603, is renowned for its transformative impact on English politics, religion, and culture. Yet, its short-lived existence – spanning only three generations – reveals a critical flaw in its reproductive strategy, which was undermined by genetic mutations and biological incompatibilities. Central to this failure was Henry VIII, whose six marriages produced only three surviving (legitimate) children – Mary, Elizabeth, and Edward – and one acknowledged illegitimate son, Henry FitzRoy, falling far short of the expectations for a dynasty that was so dependent on male heirs to secure its legacy. A compelling medical hypothesis suggests that Henry VIII's Kell-positive blood type caused obstetric complications through alloimmunisation, leading to a high rate of miscarriages and neonatal deaths, later manifested as McLeod syndrome, a rare disorder contributing to Henry VIII's physical and psychological decline. These genetic factors, combined with the Tudors' extremely limited gene pool due to consanguineous marriages, doomed their reproductive strategy.[104]

The Kell blood group system, identified in the 1940s, involves a protein antigen ('big K') present on red blood cells in about nine per cent of people of European descent. Kell incompatibility occurs when a Kell-negative mother conceives a child with a Kell-positive father. The first pregnancy *may* result in a healthy child, as the mother's immune system is not yet sensitised to the Kell antigen. However, during childbirth, miscarriage, or other events involving foetal-maternal blood mixing, the mother's immune system will make antibodies against the Kell antigen. Then, in later pregnancies, these antibodies can cross the placenta, attack a Kell-positive foetus and cause haemolytic disease of the newborn (HDN), which often leads to late-term miscarriages, stillbirths, or neonatal deaths. This pattern is the most logical explanation of the high rate of reproductive losses among Henry VIII's wives, which undermined the Tudor dynasty's ability to produce viable heirs.

Henry VIII's six marriages – to Katherine of Aragon, Anne Boleyn, Jane Seymour, Anne of Cleves, Catherine Howard, and Catherine Parr – resulted in at least thirteen documented pregnancies, with estimates suggesting up to at least seventeen when including unrecorded losses, which in my expert opinion were many. Of these, only four children survived infancy: Mary (1516, Katherine of Aragon), Elizabeth (1533, Anne Boleyn), Edward (1537, Jane Seymour), and Henry FitzRoy (1519, illegitimate, from Elizabeth Blount). This represents a seventy per cent rate of miscarriage, stillbirth, or neonatal death, far exceeding the approximately ten per cent loss rate among the pregnancies of thirty-one noblemen contemporary to Henry VIII. The obstetric histories of Katherine of Aragon, Anne Boleyn and Jane Seymour all align with the Kell alloimmunization model.[105]

Katherine of Aragon's 6–10+ pregnancies illustrate this pattern the best. Her first pregnancy in 1509 produced a stillborn daughter, followed by a son, Henry, Duke of Cornwall, in 1511, who died at 52 days. Several of her subsequent pregnancies ended in stillbirth or neonatal death, with only Mary surviving. This sequence suggests that Katherine, likely Kell-negative, became sensitised after her first pregnancy, with her antibodies attacking subsequent Kell-positive foetuses. The reason Mary survived suggests that she was a Kell-negative blood type. Anne Boleyn's four pregnancies follow a similar trajectory: her first child, Elizabeth, was born healthy in 1533, but her subsequent pregnancies ended in late-term miscarriages, consistent with sensitisation. Jane Seymour may have had as many as three pregnancies, while Henry's later wives had fewer or no pregnancies, possibly due to his declining health and perhaps impotence. This pattern supports the hypothesis that Henry was Kell-positive, potentially inherited through his maternal lineage from Jacquetta of Luxembourg, creating a major obstetric barrier to producing heirs.[106]

Jacquetta of Luxembourg (*c.*1416–1472), a prominent noblewoman from the House of Luxembourg, played a significant role in the English royal lineage through her daughter Elizabeth Woodville, who married Edward IV, producing Elizabeth of York, Henry VIII's mother. The theory that Jacquetta was a carrier of the Kell-positive blood group gene transmits this idea that she unwittingly introduced this trait into the Tudor lineage, ultimately damning Henry VIII's reproductive capabilities and his health. The Kell blood group is defined by the presence of the Kell antigen ('big K') on red blood cells, and it is present in approximately nine per cent of individuals of European descent, making it a plausible trait within a noble family like House of Luxembourg, due to their extensive intermarriage with other European members of the Peerage. The KEL gene on chromosome 7, is inherited in an autosomal codominant manner. A single copy of the K allele results in a Kell-positive phenotype (K/k or K/K), while two recessive K alleles produce a Kell-negative phenotype .

So, supposing Jacquetta was Kell-positive, she had a fifty per cent chance of passing the K allele to each of her children, including Elizabeth Woodville. This genealogical pathway – Jacquetta to Elizabeth Woodville to Elizabeth of York to Henry VIII – arguably gives us a direct route for the K allele to reach Henry, who would express the Kell-positive phenotype if he inherited even one K allele. This trait is significant for our study of Tudor reproduction because it could trigger alloimmunisation in Kell-negative mothers, and this leads us to haemolytic disease of the newborn. This condition also makes for high rates of miscarriage or neonatal death, as seen in Henry VIII's wives.[107]

Historical evidence for Jacquetta's Kell status is speculation because blood typing was unknown in the fifteenth century. However, her noble pedigree supports the plausibility of the theory. The House of Luxembourg, with familial ties to the Holy Roman Empire, French aristocracy, and Burgundian nobility, intermarried inside of a limited genetic pool, and so increasing the likelihood of rare traits like Kell-positivity. Jacquetta's first marriage to John, Duke of Bedford, didn't produce any children, but her second marriage to Richard Woodville was very prolific, creating fourteen children, suggesting that she did not face significant obstetric complications herself. In my opinion this indicates that Jacquetta was Kell-positive, avoiding sensitisation issues if her husband was also Kell-positive or if their children inherited her Kell-negative allele. The absence of any reproductive difficulties in her immediate family does not preclude her carrying the K allele, as its impact would be determined by the Kell status of her descendants' spouses.

This theory looks better and better when we examine the reproductive patterns of Henry VIII's wives, particularly Katherine of Aragon and Anne Boleyn, who both experienced a seventy per cent rate of miscarriage, stillbirth, or neonatal death across at least eleven documented pregnancies (I believe they could have had more), compared to a ten per cent loss rate among their peers' wives. If Jacquetta introduced the K allele, it would have passed through Elizabeth Woodville (fifty per cent chance) and Elizabeth of York (fifty per cent chance) to Henry VIII, who had (in my opinion) the Kell-positive phenotype, causing these terrible obstetrical complications. The suggestion that Jacquetta was the source of this trait, theoretically inherited from her Luxembourg descendants, is speculative but supported by what I view as the genetic prevalence of Kell-positivity and the Tudor reproductive record.

The House of Luxembourg's intermarriages with families like the Valois and Habsburgs provide a perfect genetic environment for the dreaded K allele's presence. The Kell hypothesis directly contradicts the sixteenth-century belief that Henry's wives were responsible for repeated miscarriages and stillbirths. In Tudor England, fertility was seen as the woman's responsibility, leading Henry to divorce Katherine of Aragon and execute Anne Boleyn for failing to produce male heirs, or worse, killing them in utero. Modern research, however, highlights male factors in recurrent pregnancy loss, including blood group incompatibilities. The high loss rate among Henry's wives, compared to their noble contemporaries, suggests that his Kell-positive status was a critical factor in the Tudor dynasty's limited reproductive capacity, undermining its ability to secure a robust lineage.[108]

Chapter 2

Legacy of the Mutant King

The Kell-positive blood type is obviously a problematic one. It caused many bad outcomes for those who carried this unlucky blood. However, there is another reason why Kell-positive blood is problematic; it can lead to a truly devastating disorder. Those who inherited this horrible disease were like fabled mortals cursed by an evil witch in some mutant version of *Beauty and the Beast*. It wrecks both the body and mind of those afflicted, in truly terrible ways. McLeod syndrome is the name of this terrible disease, a rare X-linked disorder caused by mutations in the XK gene, which is associated with the Kell-positive blood group. This condition typically manifests in Kell-positive men between ages thirty and forty, with symptoms including muscle weakness, chorea (involuntary, jerky movements), peripheral neuropathy, cardiomyopathy, and psychiatric changes such as paranoia, depression, and cognitive decline. Henry VIII, it can be argued, had all of these symptoms. The possibility that Henry VIII suffered from McLeod syndrome gives a logical explanation for his dramatic transformation from a beloved, personable young king to a cruel, paranoid, and tyrannical old monarch. Henry's 'bad blood' and resulting McLeod syndrome would have devastating consequences for the Tudor dynasty's stability and reproductive success. McLeod syndrome, as we shall soon see, presents a convincing explanation for Henry VIII's physical and mental deterioration. Historical records of Henry's life align perfectly with the symptoms of this syndrome particularly from his late thirties onward, with a notable acceleration following a severe jousting accident in 1536 at age 44.[109]

As a young man, Henry was celebrated across Europe as a 'Renaissance prince', admired for his charm, athletic prowess, musical talent, and diplomatic finesse. He excelled in physically demanding sports like jousting, wrestling, and tennis, and his musical compositions earned him praise from scholars like Erasmus. Henry could conduct complex negotiations with European powers like France and the Holy Roman Empire, earning him a well-deserved reputation as a charismatic and capable ruler. His court was a centre of intellectual and cultural activity, attracting artists, musicians, and humanists who courted his patronage. Contemporary accounts describe him as a golden boy prince, whose charm captivated foreign ambassadors and English nobles alike. Yet, by his late thirties, this image of affability began to give way to a very different reality, as chronic health issues and erratic behaviour reshaped his personality and created havoc in his reign, destabilising the Tudor court, and leaving an indelible mark on England's political, religious, and social landscape.[110]

The physical manifestations of Henry's decline began subtly but grew increasingly severe as his once idolised body was ravaged by a progressive neurological and cardiovascular disorder. Around 1527, at approximately age 36, he developed chronic leg ulcers, painful sores that persisted and worsened over time, causing significant discomfort and recurrent infections which became osteomyelitis (a really nasty bone infection) in my opinion. These ulcers, often described in contemporary accounts as foul-smelling and resistant to the rudimentary medical treatments of the time, may have started as peripheral neuropathy, a common feature of McLeod syndrome. Peripheral neuropathy is what happens when nerves are damaged – this impairs sensory and motor functions, leading to chronic pain and difficulty in moving around. The ulcers in Henry's legs not only caused physical suffering but also contributed to Henry's increasing irritability and all-around bad temper. Intense, constant pain would have exacerbated his temper, creating a vicious cycle of physical and mental stress. By 1540, Henry's physical transformation was stark: his once gloriously athletic body had succumbed to severe obesity, with armour measurements indicating a waist size of 52 inches, a dramatic departure from the lithe figure of his youth. This weight gain, coupled with his reliance on a wheelchair, hoists, and other mechanical devices for ease of mobility in his later years, indicates physical deterioration and weaknesses. He also may have had problems with breathing, or cardiomyopathy, and this is characteristic of McLeod syndrome. In fact, there are historical accounts that suggest Henry had heart palpitations and shortness of breath. These records support the presence of cardiac complications, which played a critical role in his death in 1547 at age 55. The 1536 jousting accident, during which Henry was knocked unconscious for several hours after a fall from his horse, is often cited as 'the' pivotal moment in his decline. While traumatic brain injury could account for some of Henry's neurological symptoms, like headaches, memory lapses, or personality changes, the earlier onset of leg ulcers in 1527 proves that McLeod syndrome was already well underway. The accident served as a catalyst – intensifying what was already there but not understood. The fall created a psychological crisis that demonstrably amplified Henry's behavioural changes, denoting a turning point in his reign.[111]

From a psychological perspective, Henry's behavioural deterioration had a significant impact which would change the dynamics of the Tudor court and influence England's historical trajectory for generations to come. The young king, once beloved for his courtly manners and intellectual prowess became increasingly paranoid, impulsive, and cruel, a dramatic mood shift that eroded the stability of his reign and plunged his court into a state of fear and anxiety. His ordering of the executions of Anne Boleyn in 1536 on charges of adultery and treason, Thomas Cromwell in 1540 for alleged heresy and treason, and Catherine Howard in 1542 for supposed infidelity, demonstrated a pattern of erratic decision-making and suspicion that perfectly illustrate the psychiatric disturbances of McLeod syndrome. Anne Boleyn's execution is understood to have been motivated by Henry's desire to marry Jane Seymour. The trial was a sham, with no credible evidence, marking a major shift in Henry's mental state. Now he had convinced himself that he had no limitations, and he had no compunctions about eliminating even those closest to him. The charges against Anne, including alleged affairs with multiple courtiers, were fabricated to justify her elimination, reflecting perhaps Henry's paranoia – or maybe it was enough that he wanted another wife … a younger, more fertile one? Thomas Cromwell orchestrated the execution, as a loyal advisor whose devotion to the king was absolute. He had masterminded the English Reformation, ordered the dissolution of the monasteries, and secured Henry's break with Rome. Yet Cromwell himself would not be safe from the mad king's paranoia. He was convicted on flimsy charges, demonstrating a significant breakdown in Henry's executive functioning and judgment. Thomas Cromwell's contributions to consolidating royal power and enriching the Crown through monastic wealth made his quick execution all the more shocking, highlighting the depth of Henry's cognitive decline. Henry's fifth wife Catherine Howard was executed, based on allegations of pre-contract, yet another example of this pattern, as Henry's rage, fuelled by court gossip and his own insecurities, led to the destruction of yet another tragically young wife. His rapid succession of six marriages, driven by an obsessive need to produce a male heir, clearly demonstrates emotional instability, possibly intensified by the syndrome's psychiatric effects. The psychological toll of these failures, compounded by the physical pain of his legs, exacerbated Henry's increasing volatility, as he viciously lashed out at courtiers, advisors, and even family members who failed to uphold his unmeetable expectations. The alignment of these behavioural changes with the typical onset of McLeod syndrome in middle age lends a lot of credence to the case for this diagnosis, offering us a biological explanation for the king's descent into tyranny and the chaos that engulfed his court.

The 1536 jousting accident, while significant, should not be viewed as the sole cause of Henry's decline. The physical trauma of being unconscious for hours could have caused neurological damage, potentially exacerbating symptoms like memory impairment, or cognitive decline. Contemporary sources remark upon Henry's 'migrams', mood swings, and periods of confusion following the accident, which compounded his existing symptoms in my opinion. However, Henry's leg ulcers and the gradual progression of his physical and psychological symptoms began before the accident, supporting my supposition of an underlying genetic condition. The accident acted as a catalyst, worsening the hidden neuropathy. Its timing, coinciding with Anne Boleyn's miscarriage of a male foetus in January 1536, probably served to increase Henry's psychological distress, as the loss of another potential heir deepened his obsession with his dynastic continuity. This convergence of physical trauma, reproductive failure, and genetic factors created a perfect storm, transforming Henry from a beloved monarch into a deranged madman whose actions fractured his kingdom, alienated his strategic allies, and undermined the Tudor dynasty's stability.[112]

Henry's Kell-positive blood type posed a significant immunological barrier to reproduction, causing the Tudor dynasty's high obstetrical failures. It is worth reiterating that blood group incompatibility occurs when a Kell-positive father and a Kell-negative mother produce a foetus expressing the Kell antigen, prompting the mother's immune system to produce antibodies that attack foetal red blood cells. Haemolytic disease of the newborn is a term used to describe the deadly effects of when a Kell-positive person reproduces with a Kell-negative one. The result is miscarriages, stillbirths, and neonatal deaths, particularly in subsequent pregnancies as maternal antibody levels increase. The Tudors' approximately seventy per cent pregnancy loss rate aligns with this condition, reflecting a devastating toll on their dynastic aspirations. Katherine of Aragon, Henry's first wife, endured many pregnancies, but only one child, Mary (later Mary I), surviving to adulthood, with multiple miscarriages and stillbirths, including a male heir in 1511, which I think are attributable to Kell alloimmunisation. It's possible that Mary was the only Kell-negative blood type baby, and this would explain her survival. The repeated losses took a profound emotional toll on poor Katherine, whose devout Catholic faith and determination to produce a male heir were met with heartbreak, placing a terrible strain on her marriage to Henry and setting the stage for the annulment crisis that would redefine England's religious landscape. Anne Boleyn, his second wife, gave birth to Elizabeth (later Elizabeth I) but suffered miscarriages, including a male foetus in 1536, a loss that may have precipitated her execution amid Henry's rabid desperation for a son. The miscarriage, occurring shortly after the jousting accident, intensified Henry's paranoia, as he interpreted it as evidence of divine disfavour or betrayal. Jane Seymour, his third wife, produced Edward (later Edward VI) but died shortly after childbirth in 1537. While McLeod syndrome itself does not cause infertility, its physical toll – chronic pain from osteomyelitis, Henry's reduced mobility and potential cardiomyopathy, diminished the king's reproductive capacity in his later years, particularly as his health continued its downward spiral. The psychological strain of paranoia, mood swings, and cognitive decline further destabilised his marriages, contributing to political turmoil and court intrigue that undermined the dynasty's cohesion.[113]

Henry's obsession with securing a male heir was the impetus behind monumental decisions that reshaped England's history, with repercussions that extended far beyond his reign. His annulment of his marriage to Katherine of Aragon created a permanent rift with the Catholic Church, as it led to the establishment of the Church of England through the Act of Supremacy in 1534. This schism, the result of Henry's reproductive desperation, had profound religious and political consequences, severing England's ties with Rome, confiscating monastic wealth, and intensifying domestic tensions. The dissolution of the monasteries, led primarily by Thomas Cromwell, enriched Henry's coffers but alienated traditionalists, sparking rebellions like the Pilgrimage of Grace in 1536. The executions of Anne Boleyn and her cousin Catherine Howard was provoked by suspicions of infidelity and treason, effectively demonstrating Henry's psychological instability that disrupted court cohesion. These actions alienated potential allies, weakened the dynasty's political foundation, and turned the court into a place of fear and paranoia as courtiers and advisors tip-toed around the king's volatile moods. The broader impact of Henry's health on the Tudor legacy can be seen in the religious and political machinations that followed his reign. England faced significant consequences from his break with Rome and the establishment of a Protestant monarchy under his son, Edward VI.

I would now like to introduce the hypothesis of atypical cystic fibrosis, caused by mutations in the CFTR gene, which I think provides a plausible explanation for the early deaths of several Tudor male heirs, further compounding the dynasty's reproductive challenges. Atypical cystic fibrosis, a milder form of cystic fibrosis, manifests later than classic cystic fibrosis, causing chronic respiratory infections, recurrent fevers, and, in males, infertility due to congenital absence of the vas deferens. The Tudors' practice of consanguineous marriages, a common practice among European royalty to consolidate power and secure alliances, increased the risk of homozygosity for recessive alleles, expanding the prevalence of genetic disorders. Henry VII's marriage to Elizabeth of York was intended to unite the Lancastrian and Yorkist factions after the Wars of the Roses, but it also concentrated an already narrow gene pool, creating a genetic bottleneck that heightened the likelihood of rare conditions like atypical cystic fibrosis. Similarly, Henry VIII's marriage to Katherine of Aragon, whose Spanish royal lineage was known to be the product of several generations of inbreeding, further increased these detrimental risks. Henry's older brother Arthur, Prince of Wales, died in 1502 at age 15. He was described as frail with a persistent cough which suggests a respiratory problem. His death, less than six months after his marriage to Katherine, left the Tudor succession teetering precariously, placing immense pressure on his younger brother, Henry.

To give further credence to my theory of atypical cystic fibrosis in the Tudor line is Henry FitzRoy, Henry VIII's illegitimate son, who succumbed to a wasting illness at age 17 in 1536. From all accounts it was pulmonary in nature, with symptoms of chronic coughing and weight loss, all consistent with atypical cystic fibrosis. Edward VI, Henry's only legitimate son, died in 1553 at age 15 from rapid pulmonary decline, described as 'consumption' but distinct from contagious tuberculosis. Known for being extremely contagious, tuberculosis would definitely have caused outbreaks in the crowded, unsanitary conditions of the Tudor court. Atypical cystic fibrosis is non-communicable, which aligns with the isolated nature of these deaths. The deaths of young male heirs severely weakened the Tudor line, resulting in too few successors and exposing the risks of their faulty reproductive strategy.[114]

The Tudor dynasty's reproductive strategy of relying on a single male heir per generation was terribly flawed, leaving them with severe genetic and immunological challenges. Henry VII's two surviving sons, Arthur and Henry VIII, were insufficient to secure long-term stability, particularly after Arthur's death. Henry VIII's three legitimate children, Mary, Elizabeth, and Edward – and one illegitimate son, FitzRoy – all failed to produce heirs. Edward VI, a frail boy whose reign from 1547 to 1553 was marked by political instability, died young, leaving the throne to his cousin Jane Grey who was deposed by Mary l. Mary, who reigned from 1553 to 1558, remained childless despite her marriage to Philip II of Spain, a union that created religious dissension in England and failed to produce an heir to unite the Tudor and Habsburg realms. Mary's health, plagued by chronic illnesses and false pregnancies, further limited her reproductive potential. Elizabeth, who ruled from 1558 to 1603, chose not to marry. Elizabeth I, England's iconic 'Virgin Queen', stands out as a singular female ruler in history, a queen regnant who defied the expectations of her era by choosing never to marry. This decision profoundly impacted her reign and sealed the sterile fate of the Tudor dynasty. While political strategy, diplomatic manoeuvring, and personal inclination all played roles in her choice, perhaps it was the psychological trauma of her mother Anne Boleyn's beheading by her father, Henry VIII, in 1536 that put her off marriage. This traumatic event, occurring when Elizabeth was a toddler, left an indelible mark on her psyche, fostering a deep-seated fear of marriage and its associated vulnerabilities. By remaining single, Elizabeth preserved her autonomy and safeguarded England's independence, but her decision also marked the culmination of the Tudor dynasty's failed reproductive strategy, ensuring its extinction in 1603 with her death. This event and its aftermath cannot be underestimated in how it shaped Elizabeth's view of male/female relationships.

The execution of Anne Boleyn on May 19, 1536, was a cataclysmic event in Tudor England, driven by Henry VIII's relentless quest for a male heir and his cruel, increasingly volatile temperament. Anne, Henry's second wife, had captivated the king with her intelligence, wit, and charm, prompting him to break with the Catholic Church to annul his marriage to Katherine of Aragon and marry her in 1533. This profoundly unorthodox decision, formalised through the Act of Supremacy in 1534, established the Church of England and altered the nation's religious and political future. Yet Anne's failure to produce a male heir, coupled with subsequent miscarriages including that of a male foetus in January 1536, eroded Henry's affection and trust in her fertility. Charged with adultery, treason, and incest (allegations that were fabricated to justify her removal) Anne was swiftly tried, convicted, and beheaded at the Tower of London. Her daughter, Elizabeth, then a toddler, was declared illegitimate, stripped of her title as princess, and relegated to a precarious position at court. For the young Elizabeth, who was too young to grasp the political machinations, the loss of her mother was a foundational trauma. This would be further compounded by the knowledge as she matured, that her father, the all-powerful King Henry Vlll, had ordered the execution of her mother. This event introduced a profound sense of vulnerability, shaping her perceptions of marriage, power, and personal security in ways that would define her life and reign.[115]

The psychological impact of Anne Boleyn's execution on Elizabeth ran very deep. Developmental psychology can now demonstrate that losing a main caregiver can cause children deep emotional trauma, even if they do not have clear memories of the event. Hidden or unconscious memories, such as emotional reactions, might continue to influence a person's behaviour and perspective for years to come. Elizabeth's abrupt separation from her mother, followed by her demotion from princess to 'Lady Elizabeth', would have caused her to have a deep-seated fear of abandonment and a feeling of insecurity. As she grew older, Elizabeth would find out about her mother's fate through court gossip, historical accounts, and the lingering stigma attached to Anne's name. The knowledge that her father had executed her mother for alleged infidelity, a charge inextricably linked to her failure to produce a male heir, demonstrated to Elizabeth the dangers of marriage and the precarious position of a queen consort, and more so for a queen regnant. This trauma was reinforced by subsequent events in the Tudor court: Henry's rapid remarriage to Jane Seymour just eleven days after Anne's death, the birth of Edward in 1537, which further marginalised Elizabeth, and the execution of her stepmother and kinswoman Catherine Howard, in 1542 also for charges of infidelity. These experiences taught Elizabeth that marriage was a perilous institution, fraught with betrayal, loss, and even potential death, particularly for women in positions of power. The psychological scars of her mother's beheading created a distrust of romantic entanglements, as Elizabeth came to associate marriage with the vulnerabilities that had destroyed her mother.[116]

Elizabeth's childhood and adolescence were scarred by instability and danger, adding to the impact of her mother's execution and reinforcing her distrust of marriage. Having been declared illegitimate, she spent her father's reign on the margins, living a much less prominent life than her brother Edward. Her status fluctuated with Henry's whims, and she was reinstated in the line of succession only through the Third Succession Act of 1543, a precarious position that was dependent on Henry's royal favour. The death of Henry VIII in 1547 pushed Elizabeth into a new phase of uncertainty under her brother Edward VI's reign (1547–1553). The conflicts between her Catholic sister and her Protestant brother created confusion for Elizabeth. Edward's death at age 15 in 1553 brought their half-sister Mary to the throne and her Catholic restoration posed significant risks for the Protestant Elizabeth. Rumours of Elizabeth's involvement in Wyatt's Rebellion in 1554, a Protestant uprising against Mary's marriage to Philip II of Spain, was enough for Elizabeth to be sent to the Tower of London. This was the very place where her mother had been executed years before and now Elizabeth was getting a small taste of her mother's terror. This harrowing experience, coupled with the memory of Anne's fate, must have deepened her sense of vulnerability and reinforced her distrust of marriage. The execution of her cousin, Lady Jane Grey, in 1554, and Mary's union with a Spanish husband intensified the English realm's political instability, further illustrating the dangers of marriage for a female ruler. These events, when layered on top of the foundational trauma of her mother's beheading, shaped Elizabeth's perception of marriage as a threat to a woman's personal security and agency. These things set the stage for her unprecedented decision to remain unmarried and forever childless.[117]

When Elizabeth ascended the throne in 1558 at age of 25, she faced immense pressure to marry and produce an heir, as the stability of the realm was thought to depend on a clear (male) succession. In the sixteenth century, a queen regnant was an anomaly in patriarchal society, and marriage was seen as essential to ensuring dynastic continuity and strengthening alliances. Princely suitors from across Europe vied for her hand, each representing potential diplomatic advantages for England, but also risks of unwanted foreign influence. Philip II of Spain, her late sister's husband, sought to maintain Spanish influence in England. Archduke Charles of Austria offered a tempting Habsburg alliance, while French princes Henry of Anjou and Francis, Duke of Alençon, represented welcome opportunities to counter Catholic Spanish power. Handsome and charming English suitors, such as Robert Dudley, Earl of Leicester, and later Robert Devereux, Earl of Essex, appealed to the queen and her cohort of advisers' English interests but carried their own political complications. Elizabeth, however, cleverly used her unmarried status as a diplomatic tool, engaging in prolonged marriage negotiations without committing to any suitor. Elizabeth's approach, commonly referred to as her 'marriage game', gained her and England true independence and the ability to manage powerful rivals, putting off conflicts like the Spanish Armada until 1588, when England was better prepared. However, her mother Anne Boleyn's execution left deep psychological scars, subconsciously directing Elizabeth's decision not to marry. Anne's fate proved to her daughter how deadly matrimony could be for women; it undermined her authority and relegated her to the role of broodmare.

The psychological trauma of Anne's execution was compounded by Elizabeth's awareness of her father's volatile behaviour, which transformed him from a charismatic ruler into a tyrant capable of executing two wives and numerous advisors. The knowledge that Henry VIII, the source of her paternity and royal authority, had ordered her mother's death for failing to produce a male heir would have instilled in young Elizabeth a profound distrust of men, particularly those with political ambitions. This distrust was evident in Elizabeth's relationships with her male courtiers like Robert Dudley, her longtime favourite, with whom she shared a deep emotional bond. Although Elizabeth was closely linked to Dudley, she declined to marry him, possibly due in part to the controversy over his first wife Amy Robsart's suspicious death in 1560. The parallels between Amy's death and the charges against Anne Boleyn, both involving allegations of infidelity or betrayal, may have further reinforced Elizabeth's fear of marriage, as she sought to avoid the danger that had ensnared her mother. Her later flirtations with Essex, a younger courtier whose ambitions led to his execution for treason in 1601, further suggest an emotional capacity for affection but a resolute refusal to formalise such relationships through marriage. The psychological barrier to marriage, rooted in the trauma of Anne's beheading, was intensified by these experiences, as Elizabeth carefully navigated the delicate balance between personal desire and political necessity.[118]

Elizabeth's public persona as the 'Virgin Queen' was a construct, reflecting her considered political strategy and her subconscious psychological barriers to marriage shaped by her mother's execution. By presenting herself as married to her kingdom, Elizabeth transformed her unmarried status into a symbol of devotion to England, cultivating loyalty among her subjects and deflecting criticism of her childlessness. Her speeches, such as the 1559 address to parliament, emphasised her commitment to the realm over personal desires, declaring that she was 'already bound unto an husband, which is the kingdom of England'. This kind of rhetoric reinforced her authority, allowing her to sidestep the marital expectations of a patriarchal society while maintaining her independence. The iconography of the Virgin Queen, portrayed in portraits as an ageless and nearly goddess-like figure embellished with symbols of purity and authority, reinforced her image as a monarch elevated beyond conventional matters such as marriage and procreation. Privately, however, Elizabeth's refusal to marry was deeply rooted in a subconscious fear of replicating her mother's fate. The execution of Anne, ordered by a husband who once professed love, would have taught Elizabeth that marriage could lead to betrayal, loss of power, or even death. By remaining unmarried, she ensured that no man could ever rule over her, preserving her autonomy and protecting herself from the state of marriage that had destroyed her mother.

The integration of Elizabeth's decision into the Tudor dynasty's failed reproductive strategy is central to understanding its collapse. The Tudors' reproductive efforts were plagued by a series of failures that left the dynasty with insufficient heirs to ensure continuity. Henry VII, the dynasty's founder, had two surviving sons, Arthur and Henry VIII, but Arthur's death in 1502 at age 15 placed the entire dynastic burden on Henry VIII. Henry's six marriages produced only three legitimate children – Mary, Elizabeth, and Edward – and one illegitimate son, Henry FitzRoy, none of whom produced heirs. Mary, who reigned from 1553 to 1558, remained childless despite her marriage to Philip II of Spain, a union that ignited religious tensions and failed to secure a Catholic succession. Edward VI, reigning from 1547 to 1553, died at age 15, his frail health preventing him from reaching adulthood or producing heirs. Henry FitzRoy, acknowledged as Henry VIII's son with Elizabeth Blount, died at 17 in 1536, leaving no offspring. The Tudors' reliance on a single male heir per generation, coupled with high obstetric losses and early deaths, created a precarious succession that hinged on the reproductive success of Henry VIII's children. Elizabeth's decision to remain unmarried, driven by the psychological trauma of her mother's execution, was the final blow to this fragile strategy, ensuring the dynasty's extinction with her death in 1603.

The Tudor reproductive strategy was inherently flawed, rooted in the era's patriarchal culture of male primogeniture, which prioritised male heirs and eschewed female rulers. Henry VIII's obsession with producing a male heir drove his marital and political decisions, from the annulment of his marriage to Katherine of Aragon to the executions of Anne Boleyn and Catherine Howard. The Tudor focus on a male heir, which was the fundamental factor in their beliefs about dynastic stability, impeded their ability to use female heirs for succession. Mary's rule, characterised by significant religious strife and lack of an heir, did not succeed in securing the dynasty's stability. Furthermore, Edward's premature death resulted in continued uncertainty regarding the succession. Elizabeth, the last Tudor monarch, was uniquely positioned to continue the dynasty through marriage and childbirth, but her choice to remain unmarried broke this cycle. The psychological trauma of Anne's execution, which associated marriage with danger and loss, was a critical factor in this decision. Elizabeth's awareness of her mother's fate – executed for failing to produce a male heir – intensified her reluctance to marry, as she feared a similar loss of control or betrayal. It's not a huge stretch to suggest that Henry's psychological problems associated with McLeod syndrome caused this situation to occur in the first place. The executions of other women in Elizabeth's family, such as Catherine Howard and Lady Jane Grey, and the instability of Mary's marriage to Philip II further reinforced her fears, convincing Elizabeth that marriage posed unacceptable risks to her personal security and political authority.

Elizabeth's decision to forgo marriage had profound implications for the Tudor dynasty and England's history, marking the culmination of its failed reproductive strategy. By remaining unmarried, Elizabeth avoided the risks of foreign domination, as a marriage to a Catholic prince like Philip II or a French suitor could have drawn England into continental conflicts or rekindled religious strife. Her 'marriage game' kept rival powers like Spain and France in check, as both hoped to secure an alliance through her hand, delaying hostilities such as the Spanish Armada until 1588. Domestically, her unmarried status allowed her to centralise power, fostering a cult of personality that unified the nation. The iconography of the Virgin Queen, reinforced through portraits, literature, and public appearances, presented Elizabeth as a timeless ruler devoted to her people, transcending the limitations of her gender in a patriarchal society. Her reign, spanning 1558 to 1603, was a golden age of English culture, marked by the flourishing of figures like William Shakespeare and the defeat of the Spanish Armada, achievements that cemented her legacy as one of England's greatest monarchs.[119]

However, Elizabeth's choice also created significant challenges, as the lack of a direct heir fuelled political instability and uncertainty about the succession. Throughout her reign, factions at court and in parliament pressed her to marry or name an heir, fearing that her death without a clear successor would plunge England into civil war or open it up to foreign domination. Potential rival claimants, such as Mary, Queen of Scots, and her son James VI of Scotland, posed threats to Elizabeth's authority, as did Catholic plots to restore a Catholic monarchy. Elizabeth's refusal to marry or produce an heir was a deliberate choice, but it also reflected the psychological barriers erected by her mother's execution. The trauma of losing Anne to her father's blade, reinforced by the dangers faced by other women in her family, convinced Elizabeth that marriage was too risky, both personally and politically. Her decision to name James VI as her heir in 1603, shortly before her death, resolved the succession crisis but was the end of the Tudor dynasty, as the crown passed to the Stuart line. This outcome was a direct consequence of the dynasty's failed reproductive strategy, with Elizabeth's choice serving as the final, decisive factor in its collapse.

The psychological trauma of Anne's execution shaped Elizabeth's decision in ways that intersected with the Tudor dynasty's broader reproductive failures. The dynasty's inability to produce viable heirs across generations left it dependent on Elizabeth, the last of Henry VIII's children, to secure its future. Her refusal to marry broke the dynastic chain, ensuring that no Tudor heir would succeed her. This decision was not merely a personal choice but a reflection of the dynasty's systemic weaknesses, as the Tudors' reliance on a single male heir, coupled with high pregnancy losses and early deaths, and madness caused by McLeod syndrome, created a succession crisis that Elizabeth's choice exacerbated.

Elizabeth never publicly spoke about her mother, but subtle acts – such as wearing a locket ring with Anne's portrait inside of it – hint at a nuanced connection to her memory, mingling sorrow with a discreet acknowledgment of her mother's legacy. Anne Boleyn's execution was not just a personal tragedy for Elizabeth but a symbol of the dangers inherent in patriarchal regency which prioritised male heirs at the expense of dynastic resilience. Elizabeth's choice to remain unmarried, while strategically brilliant in preserving her agency and England's independence, was also a deeply personal response to the trauma of her mother's death. By refusing to marry, she avoided the vulnerabilities that had destroyed Anne, but she also ensured that the Tudor dynasty would end with her, a poignant conclusion to a family plagued by reproductive failure.

In conclusion, Elizabeth I's decision to remain unmarried was a singular act of agency, profoundly influenced by the psychological upheaval of her mother Anne Boleyn's beheading by her father, Henry VIII. This early loss, occurring when Elizabeth was just 2^{1}/2 years old, instilled a deep-seated fear of vulnerability and betrayal, reinforced by the executions of other women in her family and the instability of the Tudor court. The knowledge that marriage could lead to loss of power, personal danger, or even death – exemplified by her mother's fate – deterred Elizabeth from entering a union that could compromise her autonomy.[120] By crafting the persona of the Virgin Queen, she transformed her unmarried status into a source of strength, using it to maintain England's independence, balance European powers, and unify her realm.[121] Yet, this decision also sealed the Tudor dynasty's fate, marking the culmination of its failed reproductive strategy. The dynasty's reliance on a single male heir, coupled with its inability to produce viable successors, left it dependent on Elizabeth, whose trauma-driven choice to forgo marriage ensured its extinction in 1603. Elizabeth's legacy as one of history's greatest monarchs is inseparable from the psychological impact of her mother's execution, a trauma that shaped her reign and brought the Tudor dynasty to its poignant end. Her decision to remain the 'Virgin Queen' preserved her authority and England's independence but sealed the dynasty's fate, marking the end of the Tudor line. The Tudors' rigid adherence to male primogeniture, a cultural norm prioritising male inheritance, limited their ability to leverage female rulers for dynastic continuity, unlike their European counterparts. The combination of Kell incompatibility, potential cystic fibrosis, and a narrow gene pool created a reproductive strategy doomed to collapse, culminating in the dynasty's extinction in 1603 with Elizabeth's death and the succession passing to the Stuarts through James VI of Scotland, who became James I of England.

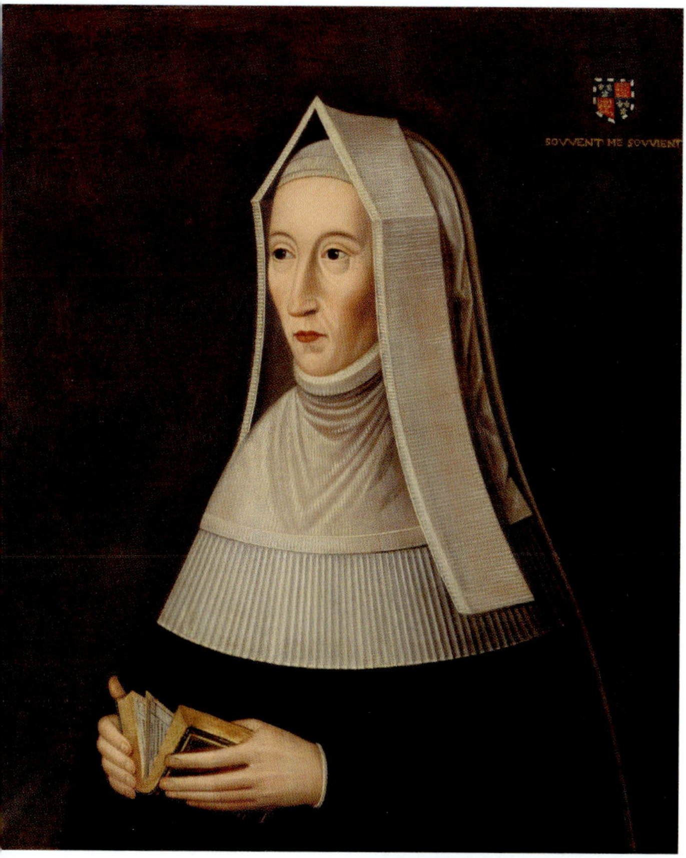

Sixteenth-century painting of Margaret Beaufort in prayer, by Meynnart Wewyck. (Public domain)

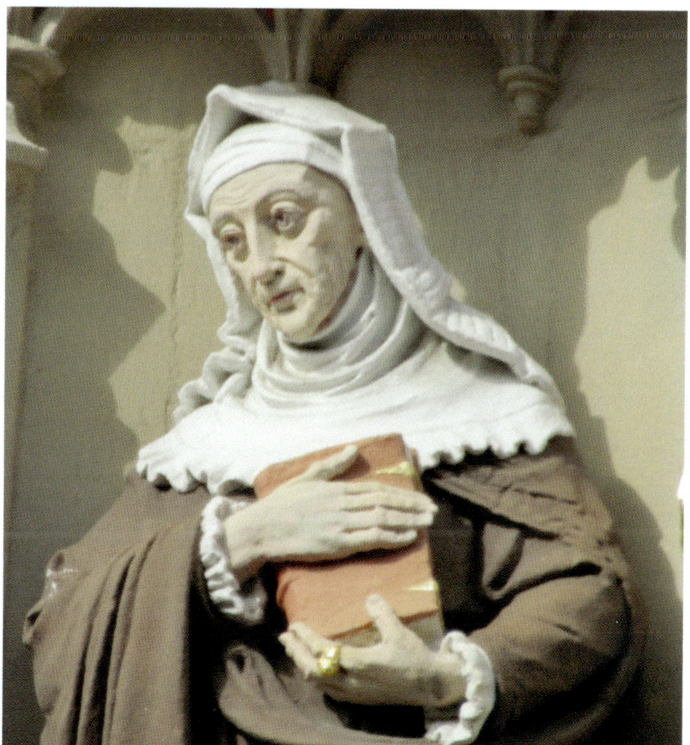

Margaret cultivated an image of holiness especially in the last decades of her life. (Public domain)

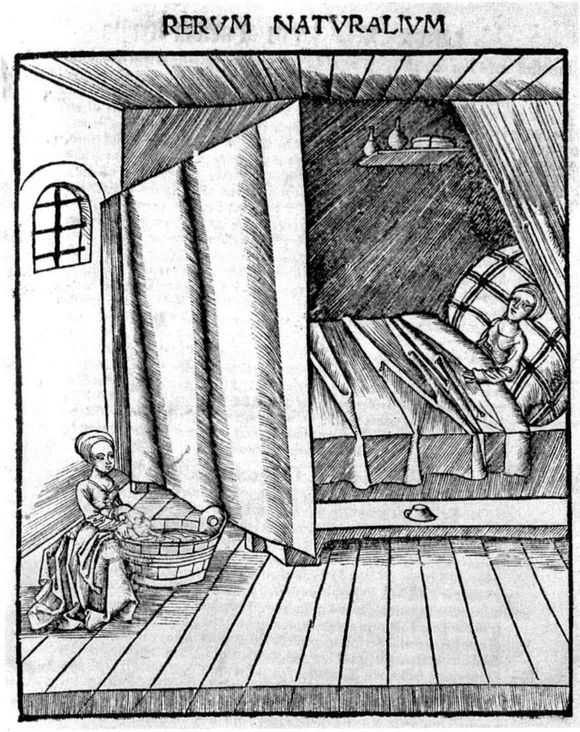

Sixteenth-century woodcut depiction of a woman with her midwife bathing the newborn. (Public domain)

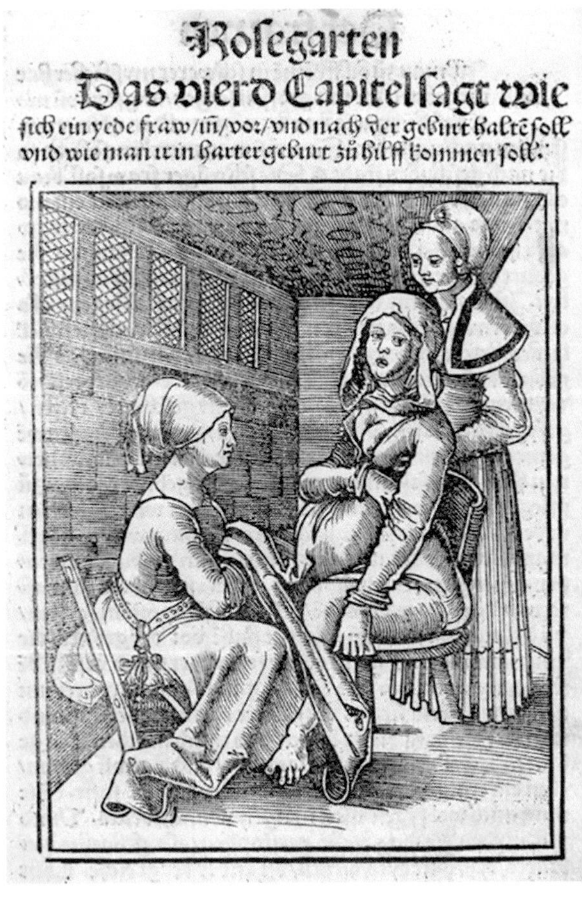

Childbirth scene from the sixteenth-century midwifery handbook *The Byrth of Mankynde,* complete with birthing stool. (Public domain)

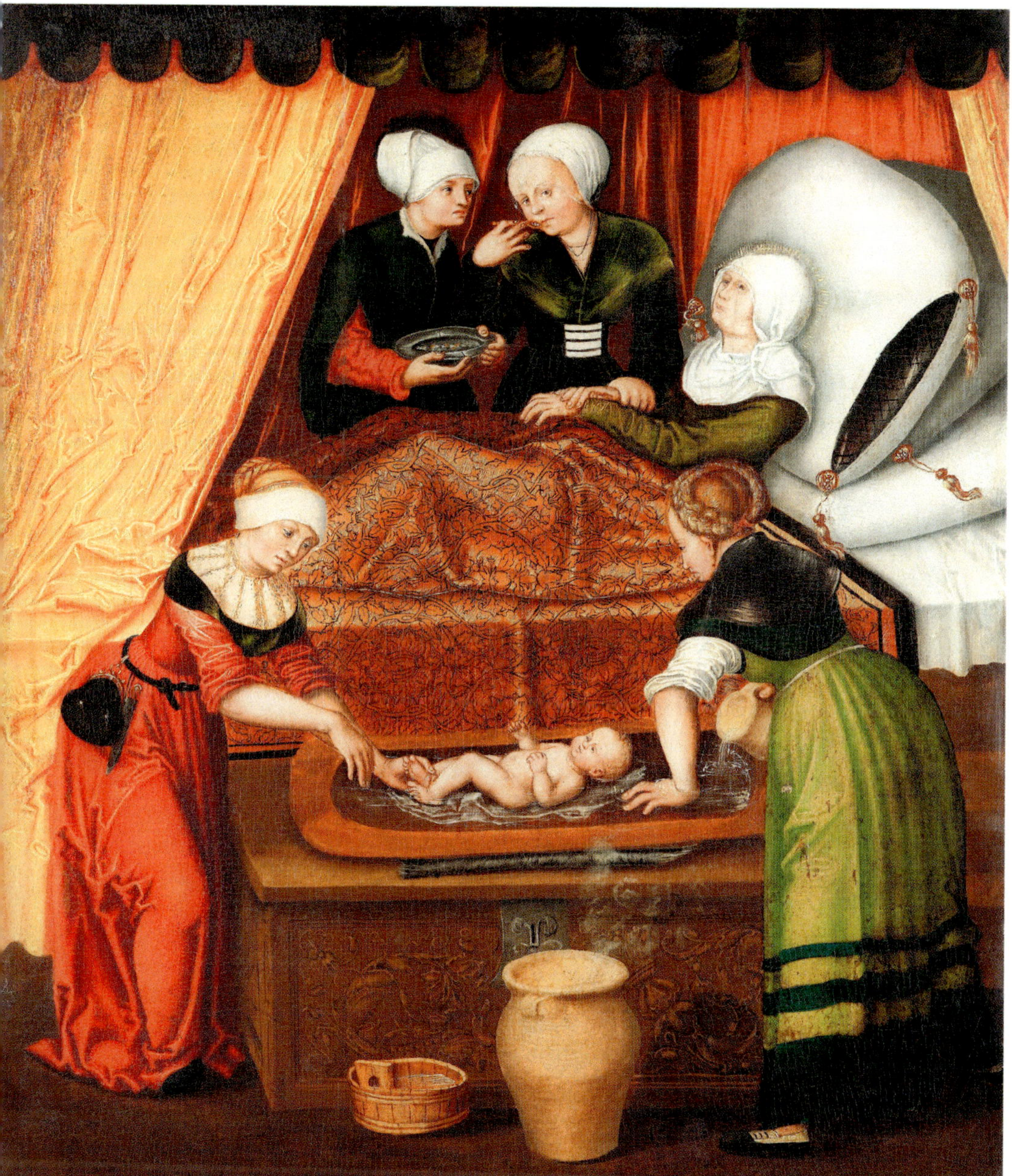

*The Birth of John the Baptist c.*1518 by Lucas Cranach the Elder. (Public domain)

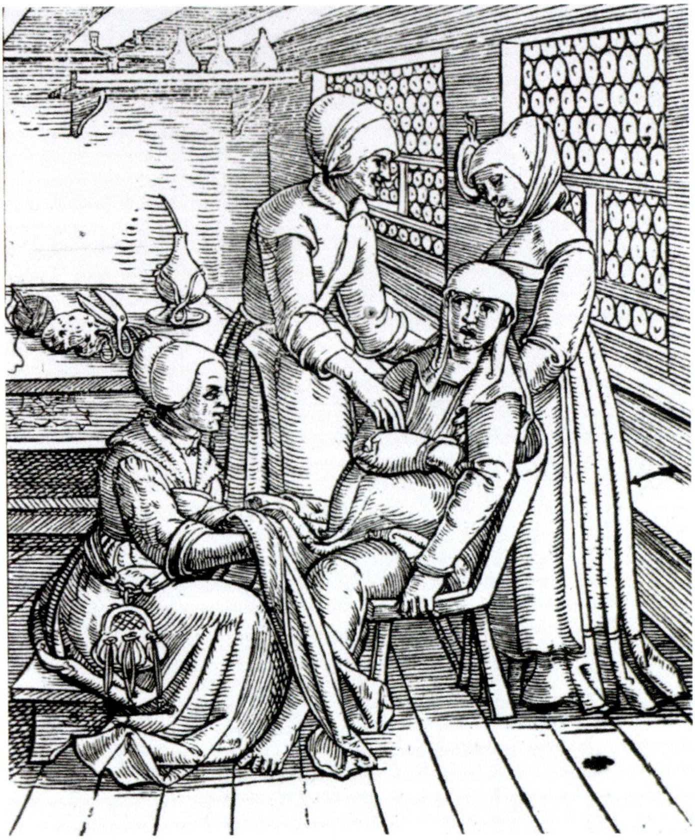

Sixteenth-century woodcut of three midwives attending a birth. (Public domain)

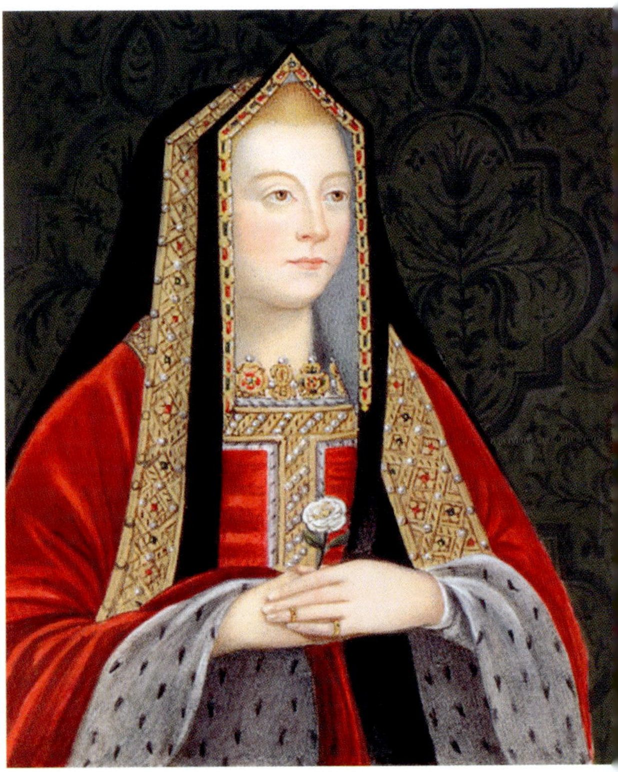

Elizabeth of York holding the white rose of York. (Public domain)

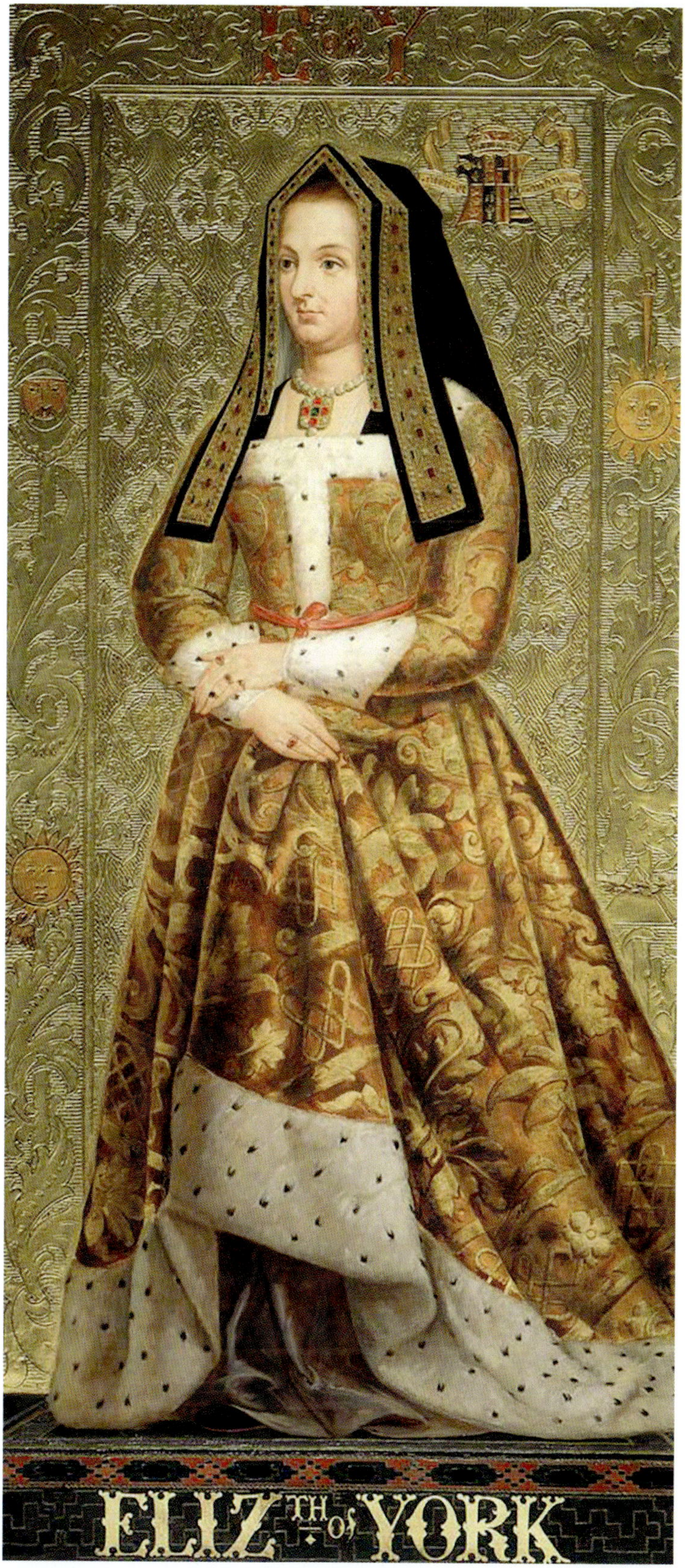

Full-length portrait
of Elizabeth of York.
(Public domain)

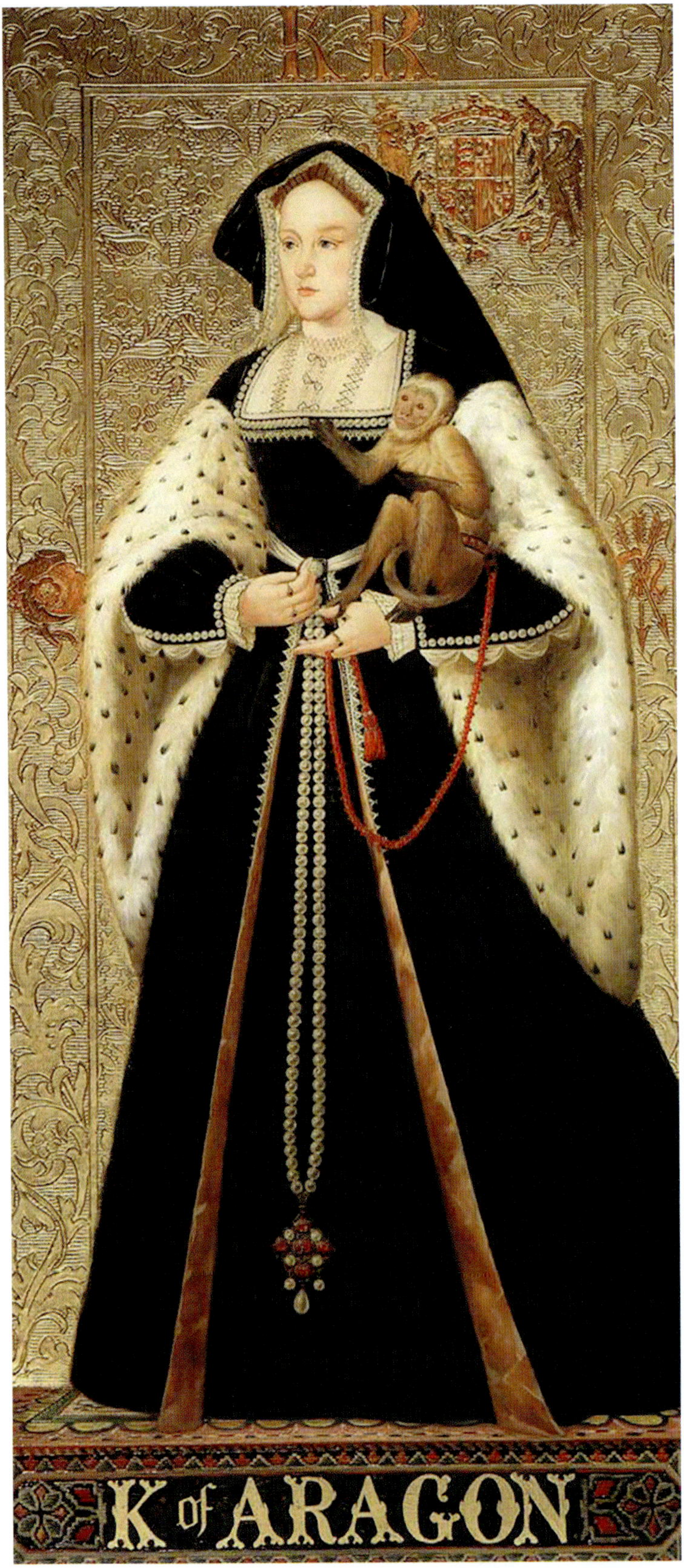

Full-length portrait of young queen consort, Katherine of Aragon. (Public domain)

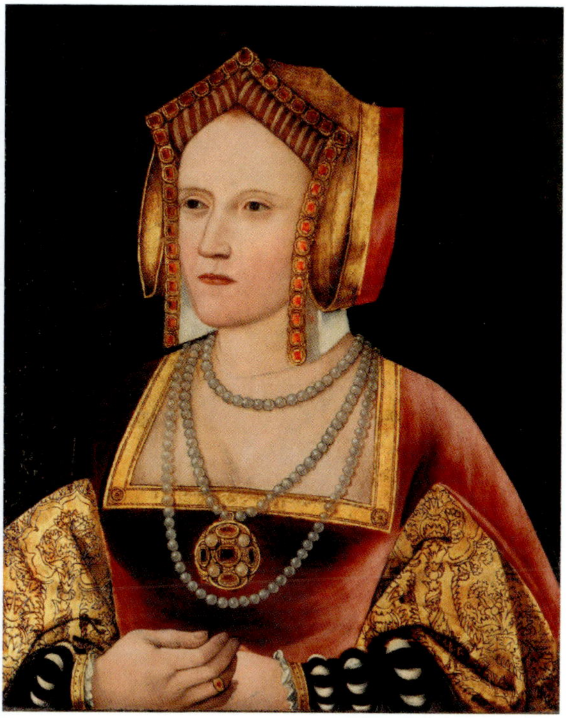

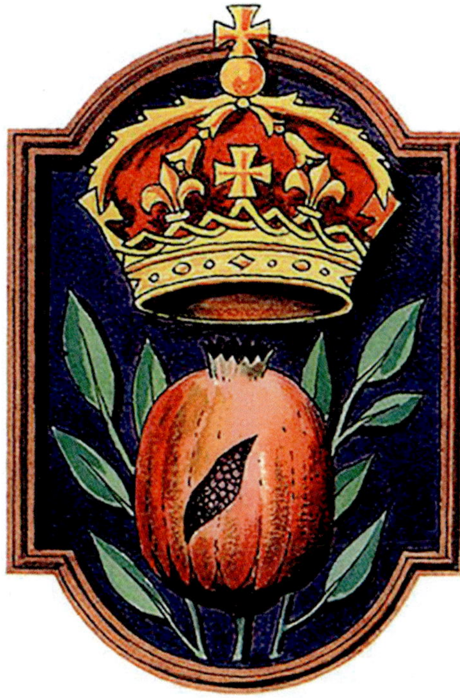

Above left: Katherine of Aragon in her prime, *c*.1520, before the Great Matter arose. (Public domain)

Above right: The badge of Katherine of Aragon; the pomegranate symbolises fertility. (Public domain)

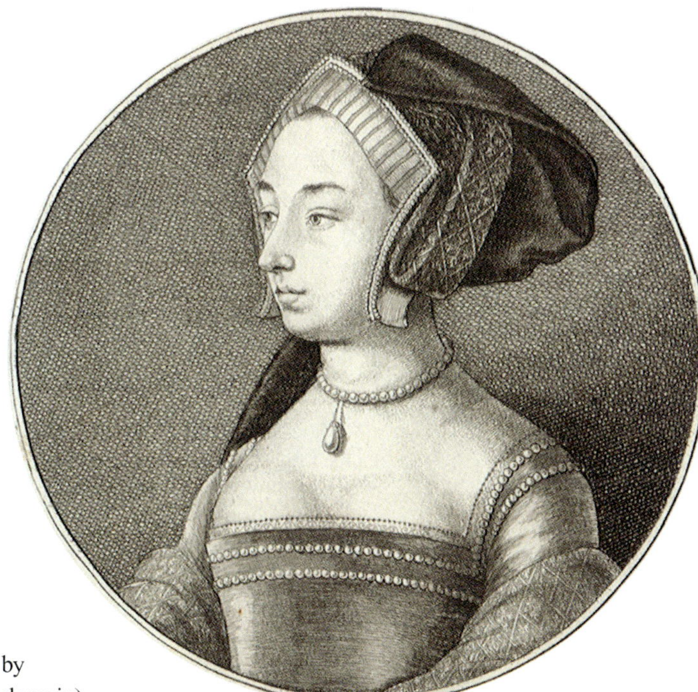

Anne Boleyn *c*.1530–1536 by Wenceslaus Holler. (Public domain)

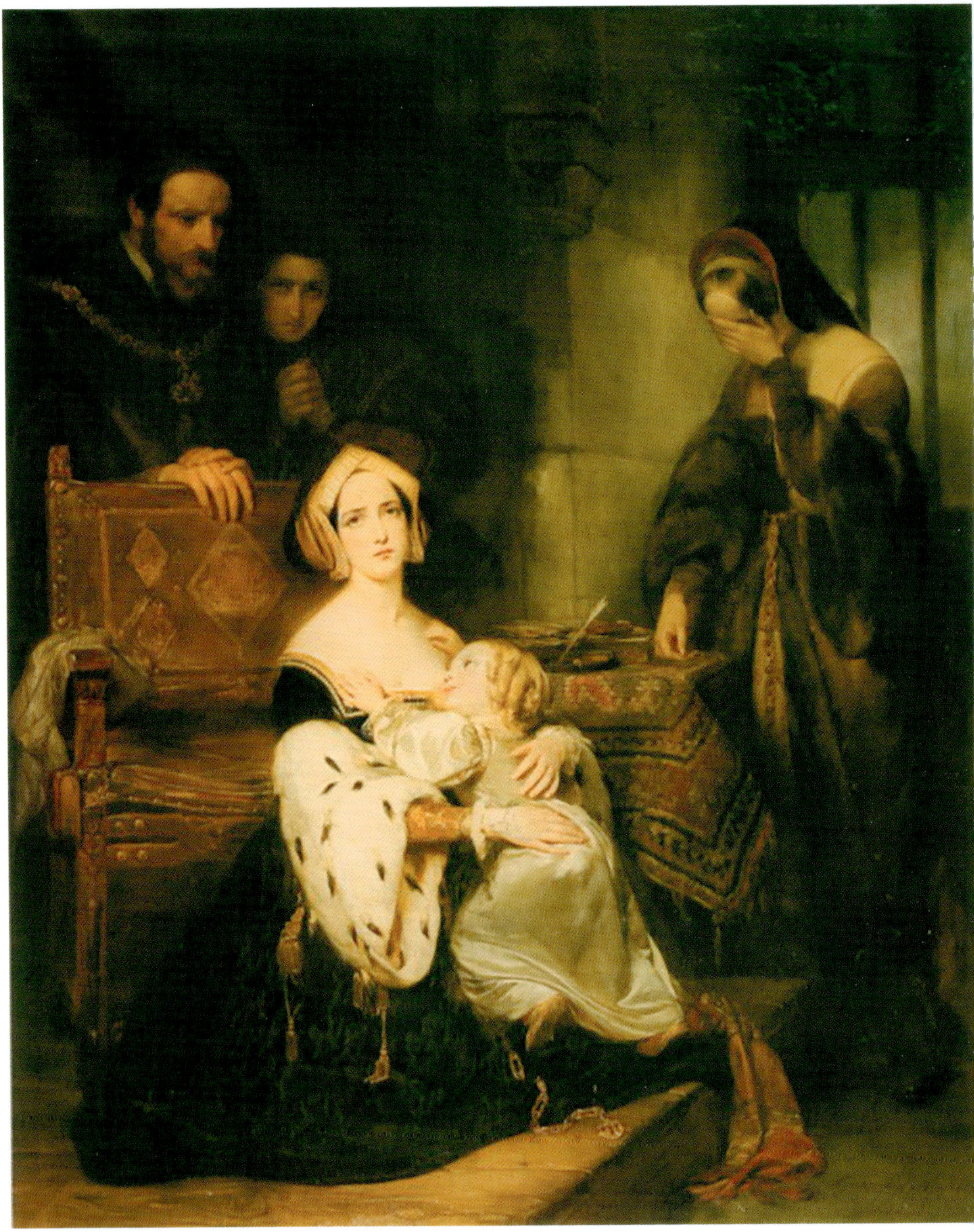

Nineteenth-century depiction of Anne Boleyn saying goodbye to her daughter, Princess Elizabeth, by Gustave Wappers. (Public domain)

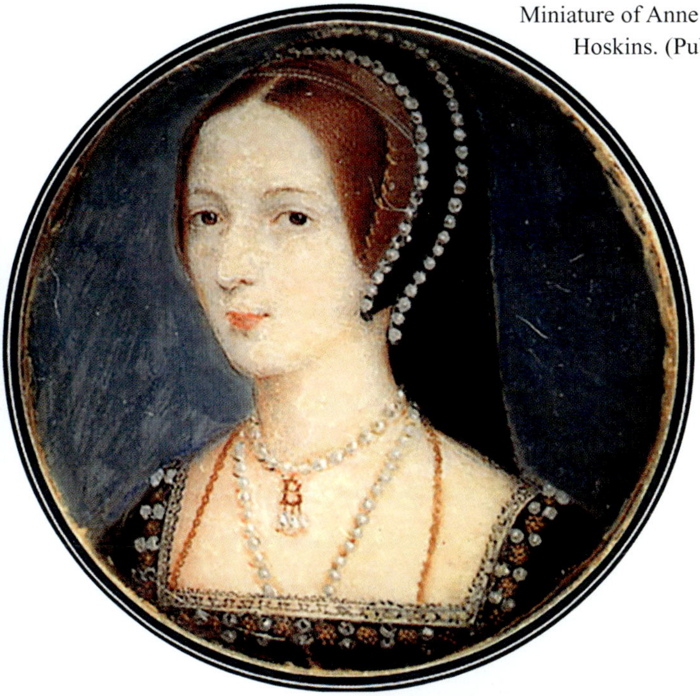

Miniature of Anne Boleyn, attributed to John Hoskins. (Public domain)

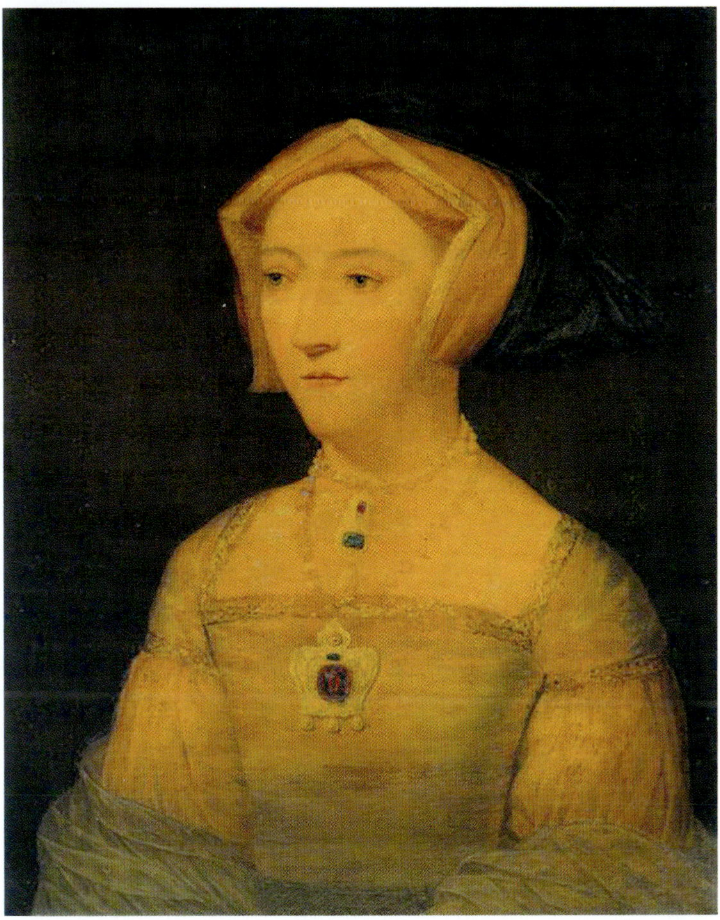

Hans Holbein portrait of Jane Seymour. (Public domain)

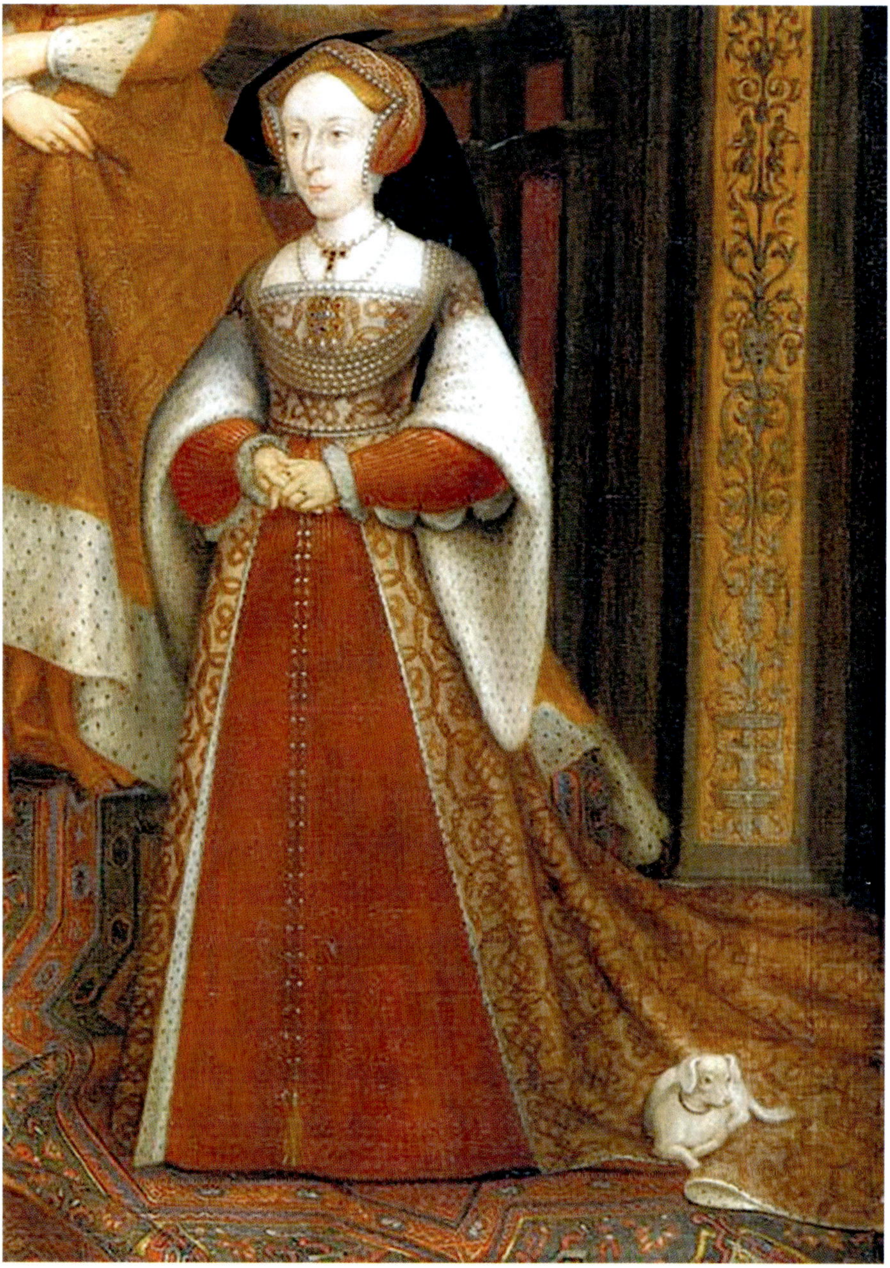

Jane Seymour, Whitehall Dynasty Mural of Henry VIII by Hans Holbein. (Public domain)

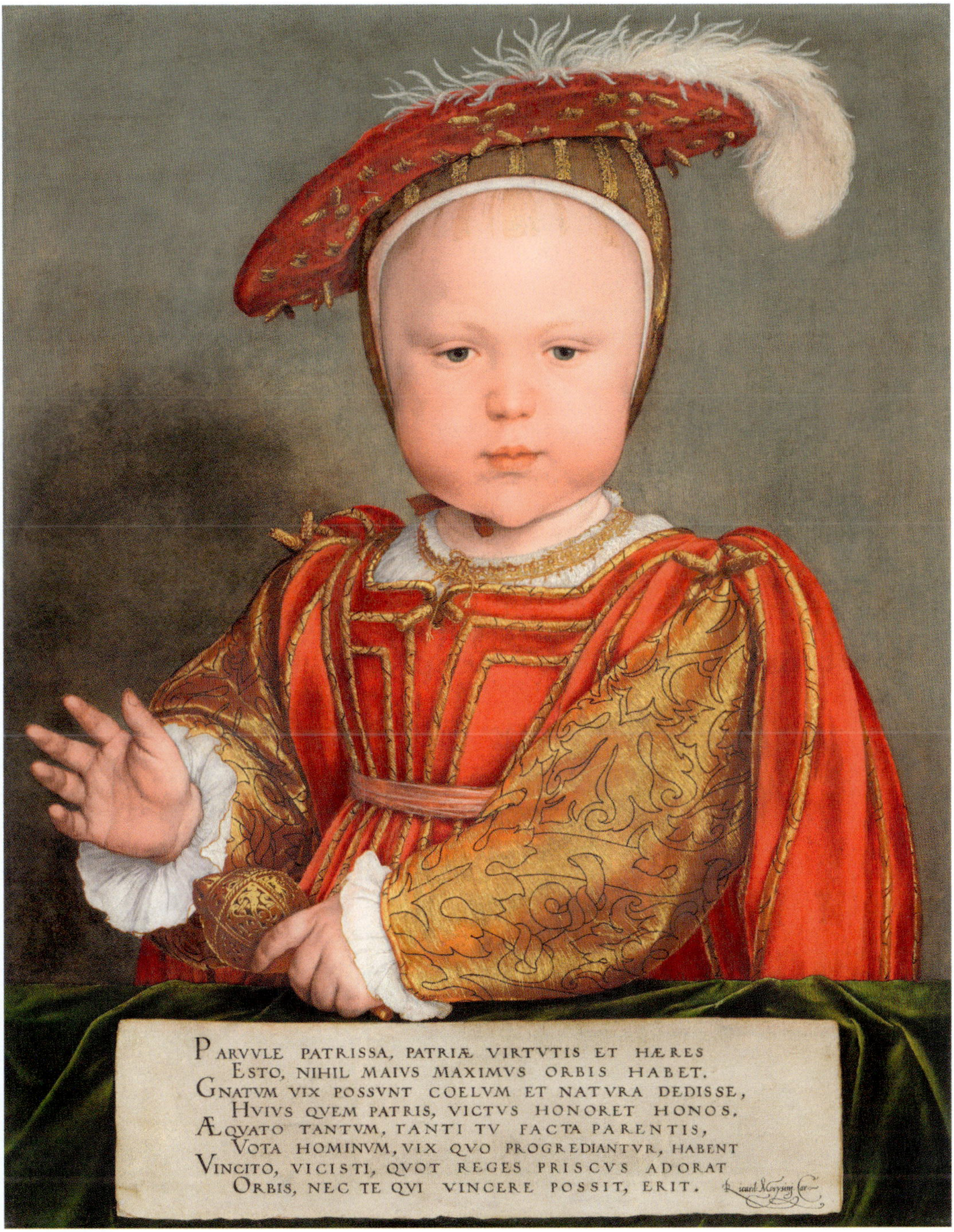

Baby Prince Edward VI by Hans Holbein, *c*.1538. (Public domain)

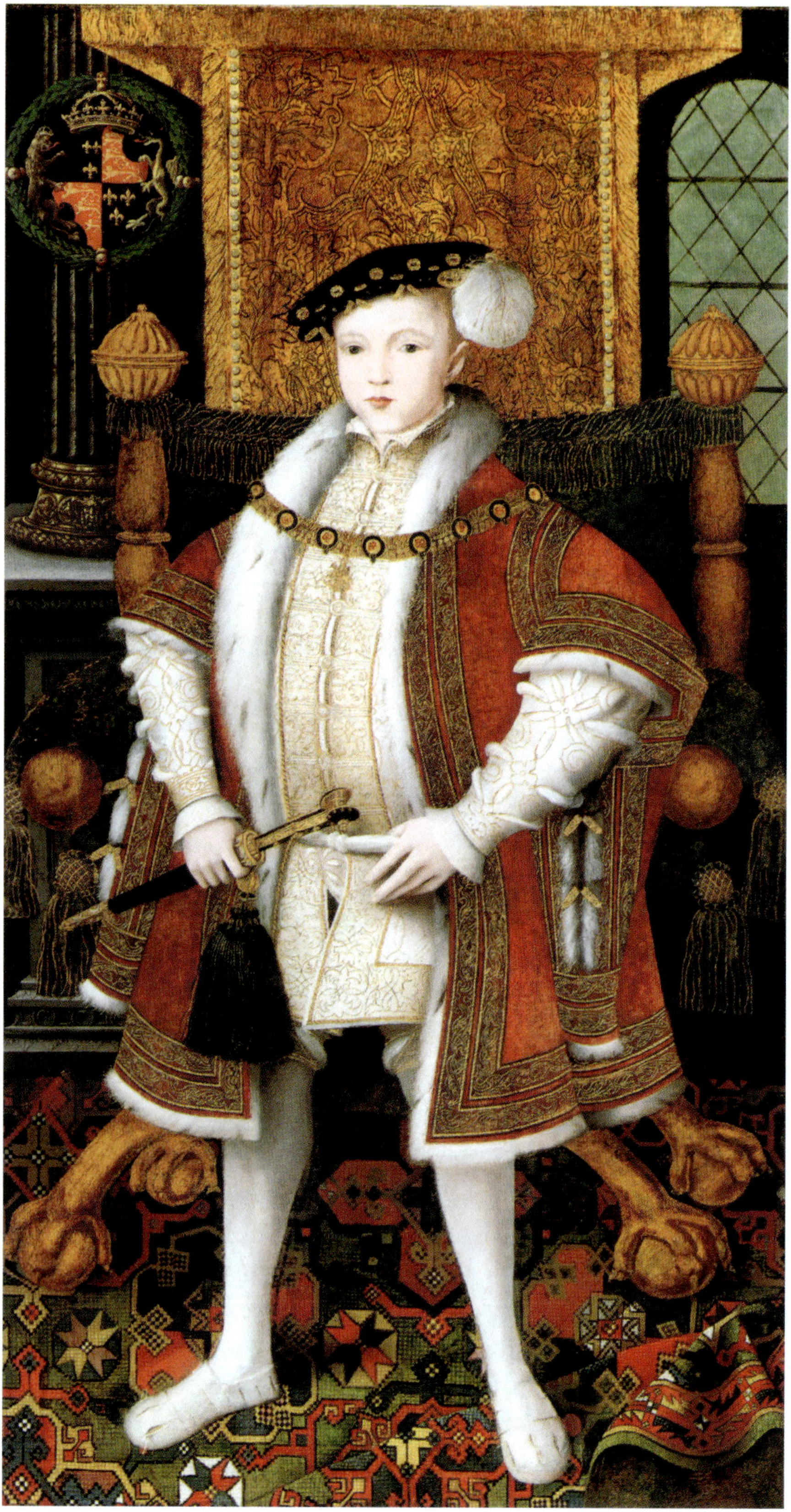

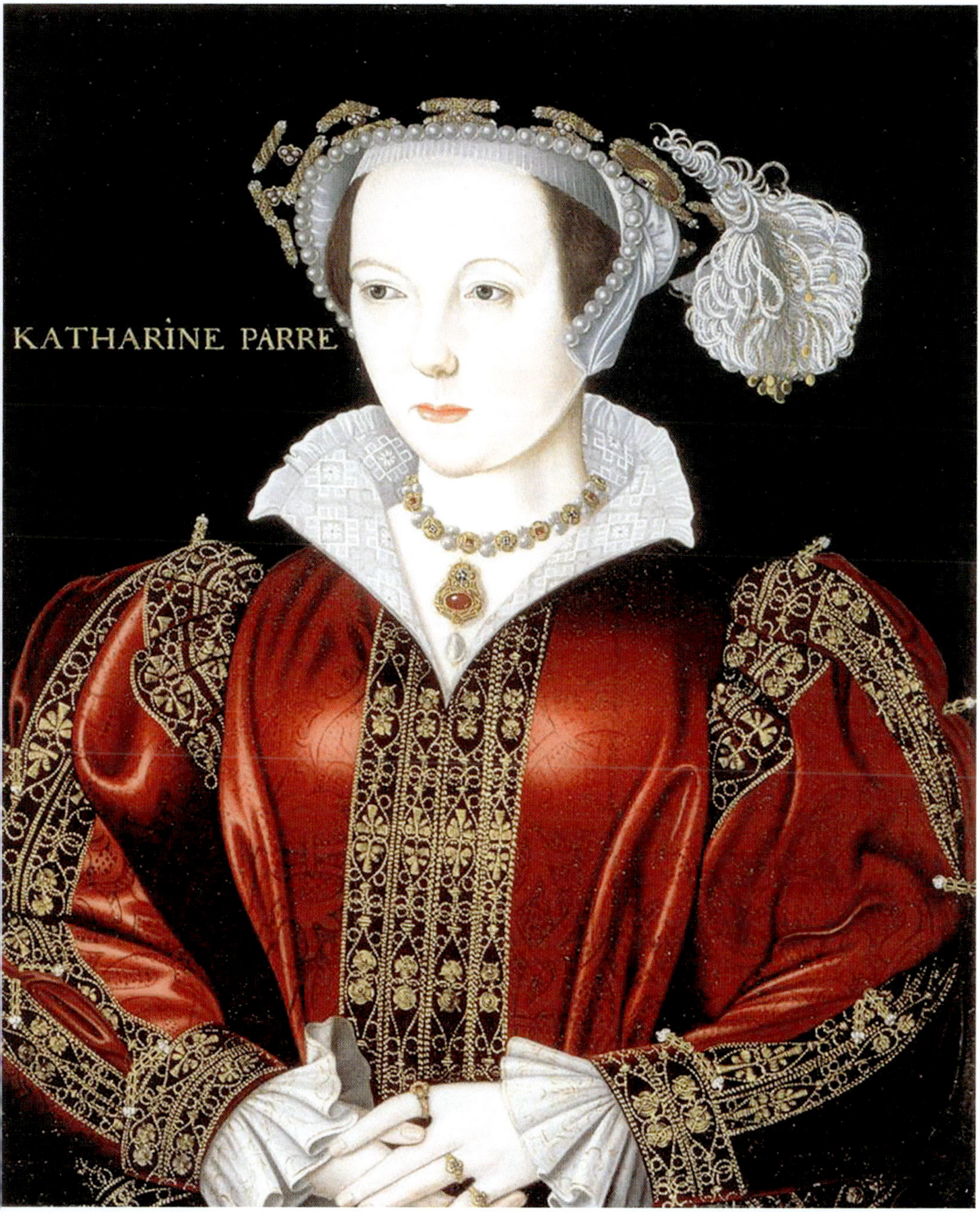

Above: Catherine Parr, sixth wife of Henry VIII. Artist unknown. (Public domain)

Opposite: Edward VI (1537–53), *c*.1547. Unknown artist, now attributed to 'Workshop associated with Master John'. (Public domain)

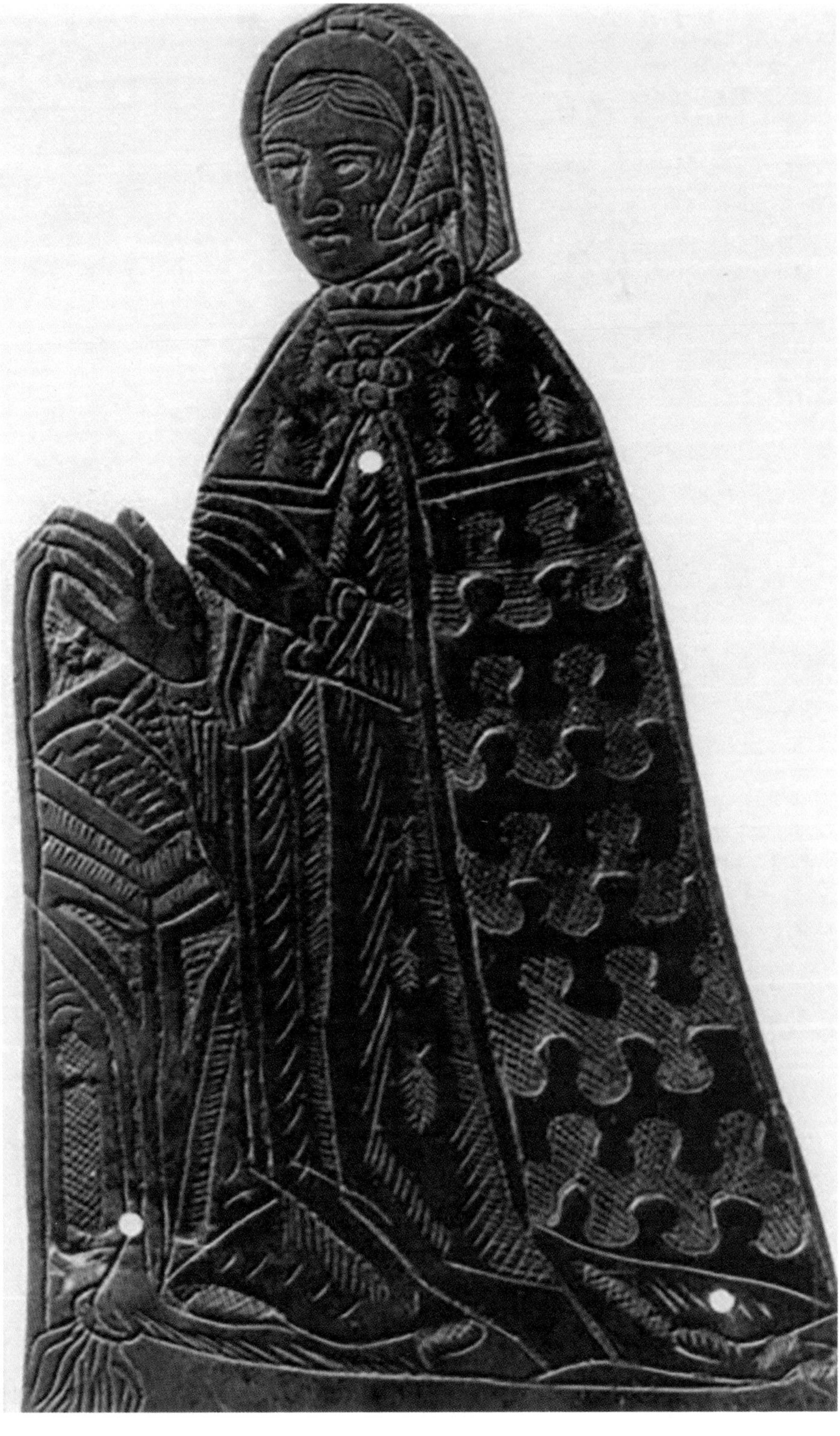

Memorial brass of Elizabeth 'Bessie' Blount. (Public domain)

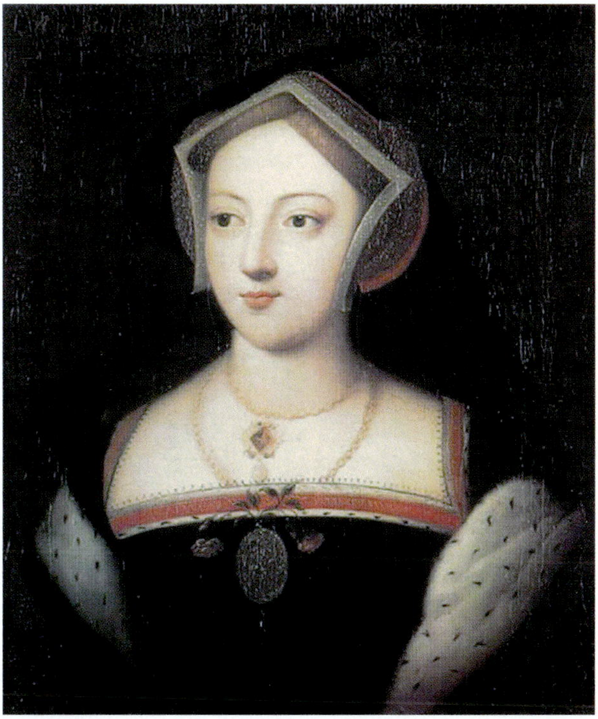

Right: Eighteenth-century depiction of Mary Boleyn. Artist unknown. (Public domain)

Below: Woodcut depicting a witch burning. (Public domain)

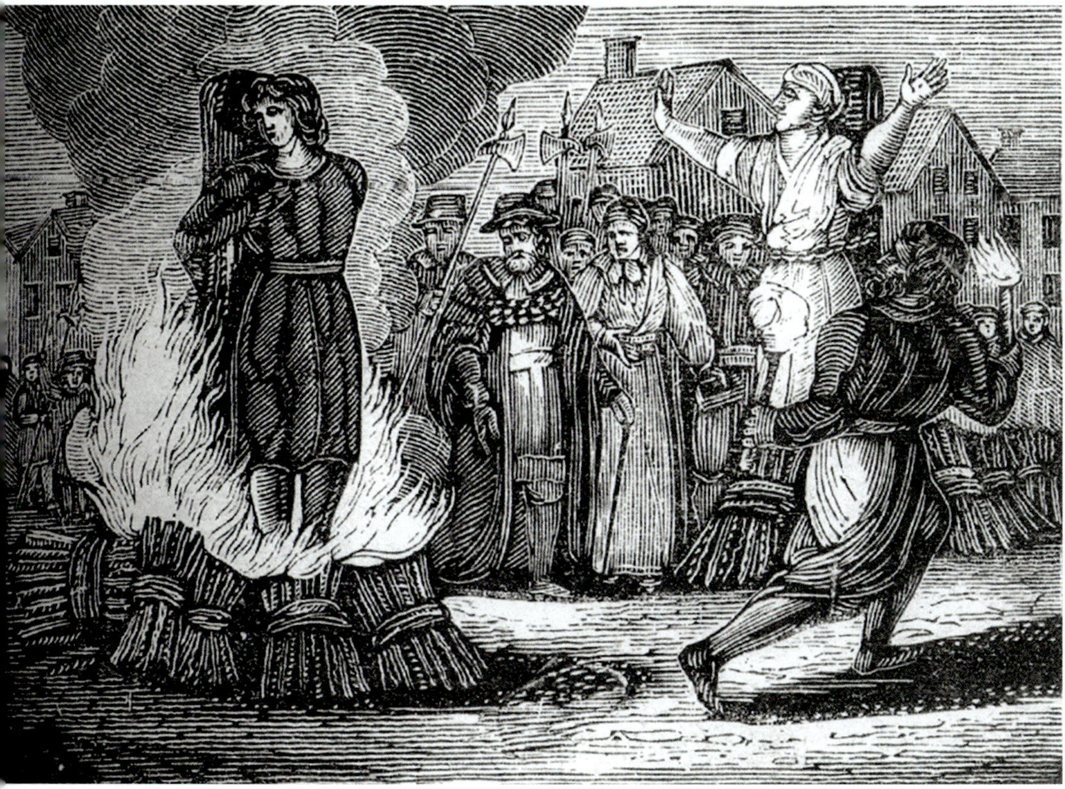

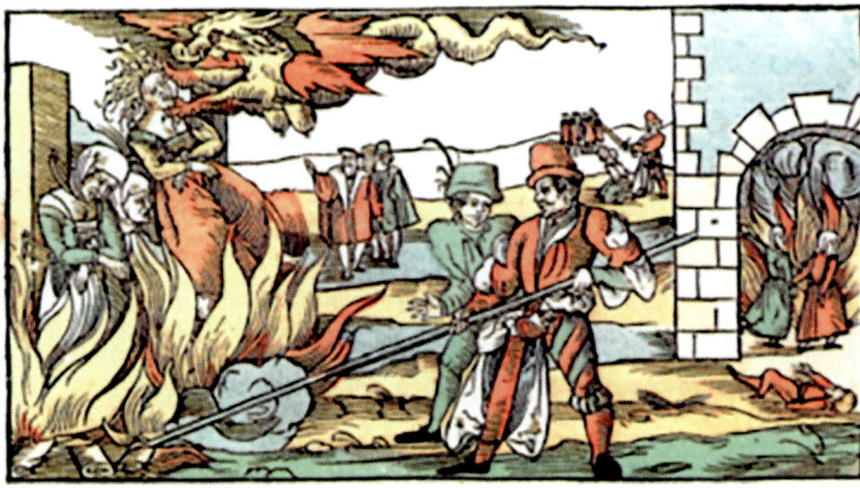

Fifteenth-century engraving of women burning at the stake. (Public domain)

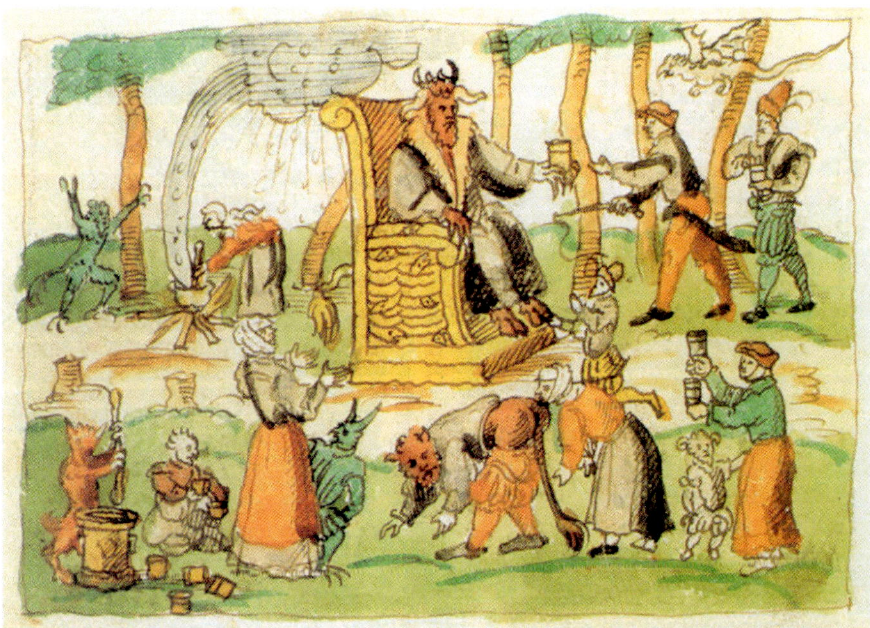

The Witches' Sabbath. Chronicle by Johann Jakob Wick (sixteenth century). (Public domain)

Chapter 3

Dynastic Stagnation Versus Dynastic Proliferation

In stark contrast to the Tudors, the Habsburg dynasty dominated Europe from the thirteenth to the twentieth centuries and achieved remarkable longevity through a well-organised multi-branch structure, prolific reproduction, and strategic adaptability. This is a powerful alternative to the Tudors' failed dynastic success. The Tudors pinned their hopes on a single male line, but the Habsburgs created a decentralised dynastic network, with branches of this great family ruling Austria, Spain, the Holy Roman Empire, and other territories. This structure ensured that the failure of one line did not wipe out the whole dynasty, which created a resilience that allowed them to weather genetic, political, and military challenges. Emperor Charles V, who ruled from 1516 to 1556, oversaw a vast empire spanning Europe, the Americas, and parts of North Africa, famously described as one 'on which the sun never sets'. His four legitimate children, including Philip II, continued the Spanish Habsburg line, while his brother Ferdinand I sustained the Austrian branch. Maximilian II and Rudolf II are the children from his Bohemian line. When the Spanish lineage ended with Charles II's death in 1700, the Austrian branch continued, eventually turning into the Habsburg-Lorraine dynasty under Maria Theresa, who ruled from 1740 to 1780. This redundancy allowed the Habsburgs to bounce back after the death of its rulers, the perfect example being Charles V's grandson Don Carlos in 1568, who suffered from severe physical and mental disabilities due to inbreeding. Don Carlos was unfit to rule, mandating his confinement and eventual death under mysterious circumstances.[122]

The Habsburgs' highly prolific marriages were essential to their reproductive successes and the overall health of their dynasty, minimising the risks of infant mortality and the genetic disorders that plagued so many royal families. Philip II, king of Spain from 1556 to 1598, married four times, producing eight children, including Philip III, who continued the Spanish line. Despite the sad death of his son Don Carlos and, tragically, several other children from his first wife, Maria Manuela of Portugal, the sheer number of pregnancies increased the likelihood of some surviving children. Maria Manuela, herself a product of a consanguineous marriage between Portuguese and Spanish royalty, bore Don Carlos. His disabilities ranged from epilepsy to violent outbursts, beautifully exemplifying the risks of inbreeding. Philip's later marriages to Elisabeth of Valois and Anna of Austria ensured the continuation of the Spanish Hapsburg line. Similarly, Ferdinand I and his wife, Anna of Bohemia and Hungary, had fifteen children, giving the dynasty a nice, robust pool of offspring stretching across the Austrian branch. Their children, including Maximilian II and Archduke Ferdinand, strengthened the dynasty's hold on Central Europe, securing territories like Bohemia and Hungary against Ottoman invasions. This prolific creation of heirs contrasts sharply with the Tudors' limited pregnancies, where Henry VIII's six marriages only had three surviving legitimate children, a meagre offering that left the dynasty vulnerable to extinction. The Habsburgs' strategy of encouraging multiple marriages and pregnancies across branches diluted the impact of specific immunological diseases, such as Kell incompatibility, which crippled the Tudors' reproductive success.

Maximilian I's marriage to Mary of Burgundy in 1477 brought the wealthy Burgundian Netherlands into Habsburg control, a fabulous acquisition that increased their economic power and provided a solid foothold in Western Europe. The Burgundian inheritance included prosperous cities like Antwerp and Bruges, which helped increase the Habsburgs' wealth that enabled their military campaigns. These military successes added to their status as a towering European power. Their son, Philip the Handsome, married Joanna of Castile, uniting the Spanish and Habsburg lines and produced Charles V, future Holy Roman Emperor, whose reign some historians believe marked the zenith of Habsburg influence.[123]

These marriages expanded territorial holdings and, to some extent, mitigated the effects of inbreeding by introducing desperately needed fresh genes, although consanguinity remained a continual challenge. For example, Charles V's marriage to Isabella of Portugal, his first cousin, produced Philip II. Then Philip II's marriage to Elisabeth of Valois, brought in French royal blood thus enlarging the gene pool while creating an alliance with France – a double win. The Habsburgs' marriage strategy was not just about territorial acquisition but also about creating alliances that strengthened their position against formidable France, the fearsome Ottoman Empire, and later the Protestant states of Northern Europe. In contrast, the Tudors' more insular marriages, such as Henry VII's to Elizabeth of York and Henry VIII's to Katherine of Aragon, reinforced a narrow gene pool, amplifying the risk of recessive disorders and limiting their diplomatic reach. The Tudors' failure to forge extensive marriage alliances left them isolated, particularly after the break with Rome, which alienated Catholic Europe and restricted their ability to secure foreign support.

The Habsburgs' willingness to accept female rulers under certain circumstances further enhanced their dynastic resilience, a flexibility Henry VIII would not abide. Maria Theresa's reign from 1740 to 1780 beautifully exemplifies this adaptability, demonstrating how female power could sustain a dynasty under pressure. Her marriage to Francis of Lorraine produced sixteen children, including Marie Antoinette, ensuring dynastic continuity through the Habsburg-Lorraine line. Maria Theresa's reforms, including modernising the Austrian administration, strengthening the military, and expanding education, solidified her legacy, showing how queens could build and even enhance dynastic stability. Her ability to manage complex alliances, such as the Diplomatic Revolution of 1756, which aligned Austria with France against Prussia, is one great example of her sharp intellect and political savvy.[124] This openness to female succession, particularly in the Austrian branch, provided a fallback when male heirs were scarce, a strategy Henry VIII wanted to avoid. Elizabeth I's decision not to marry, while politically strategic in maintaining her independence and avoiding foreign domination, ended the Tudor line, highlighting their inability to adapt to reproductive challenges. Elizabeth's choice may have been influenced by the instability of her father's marriages, the execution of her mother, Anne Boleyn, or the dynasty's troubled reproductive history, but ultimately it left England without a Tudor heir.

Genetically, the Habsburgs faced significant challenges due to their practice of consanguineous marriages, most notably in Charles II of Spain, whose severe physical and mental disabilities were a direct result of extreme inbreeding. His parents, Philip IV and Mariana of Austria, were uncle and niece, resulting in an inbreeding coefficient of 0.25, equivalent to the offspring of siblings. This led to conditions like mandibular prognathism (the 'Habsburg jaw'), a devastating facial deformity caused by recessive alleles, and infertility, which ended the Spanish line. His inability to produce an heir sparked the War of the Spanish Succession (1701–1714), a conflict that reshaped European alliances and marked the abrupt end of the Spanish Habsburgs. However, the Habsburgs' multi-branch structure enabled the dynasty to survive an otherwise devastating problem. While the Spanish line failed, the Austrian branch continued under Emperor Charles VI, whose daughter Maria Theresa ensured the dynasty's survival through the Habsburg-Lorraine line.[125] The Tudors, in contrast, had no such fall-back lineages, with their entire dynasty resting on Henry VIII's limited progeny, leaving them fatally vulnerable to the cumulative effects of genetic disorders like Kell incompatibility and atypical cystic fibrosis.

The Habsburgs' political and cultural cultivations complemented very well their reproductive strategy, enabling them to successfully navigate the complex dynamics of European power across centuries. They maintained a vast network of alliances through marriages, diplomacy, and military campaigns, ensuring their influence across Europe. Charles V maintained his empire through strategic marriages and support from regional leaders, including German princes and Spanish nobles. His abdication in 1556 divided up the empire between his son Philip II (Spain and its colonies) and brother Ferdinand I (Austria and the Holy Roman Empire), shows foresight, ensuring the dynasty's long-term survival.[126] Philip II's marriage to Mary I of England, though childless, briefly aligned England with the Habsburgs, highlighting their ability to amass power beyond their core territories. The marriage, part of Philip's broader strategy to counter French influence, illustrates the Habsburgs' use of dynastic unions to shape European politics to their advantage even if the union ultimately failed to produce an heir. The Habsburgs also manoeuvred the Protestant Reformation with a blend of Catholic orthodoxy and very pragmatic alliances, maintaining their influence despite religious upheavals. Ferdinand I's negotiations at the Peace of Augsburg in 1555 established a framework for religious coexistence in the Holy Roman Empire, balancing Catholic interests with the Protestants and so preventing the empire's fragmentation. His successors, like Rudolf II, faced challenges from religious tensions but maintained Habsburg dominance through diplomacy and cultural patronage, nurturing a vibrant court in Prague that rivalled the intellectual centres of Renaissance Europe.[127]

The Habsburgs' economic blueprints enhanced their dynastic resilience, providing the resources needed to sustain their extensive empire. The wealth from the Spanish colonies, particularly silver from mines in Mexico and Peru, bankrolled Spain's military campaigns and diplomatic efforts under Philip II, despite the economic strain of prolonged wars.[128] The Austrian Habsburgs, meanwhile, utilised the agricultural and commercial resources of Central Europe, particularly in Bohemia and Hungary, to fund their defence against Ottoman aggression. This economic adaptability contrasts with the Tudors' more limited financial base, which relied heavily on reappropriated monastic wealth and domestic taxation, a poor strategy for long-term dynastic stability. Henry VIII's dissolution of the monasteries did give him a temporary windfall, but the lack of a diversified economic plan and the costs of his military campaigns, such as the invasions of France and Scotland, strained the royal finances, thus severely limiting the Tudors' ability to project power or secure alliances.

There are numerous examples of the Habsburgs' resilience and ability to recover from setbacks, a quality that set them miles apart from the Tudors. The death of Don Carlos in 1568, a potential heir to Philip II, was a significant blow, but Philip's subsequent marriages to Elisabeth of Valois and Anna of Austria produced other heirs, thus securing continuity in the Spanish line. The loss of Don Carlos, while a tragedy, did not derail the dynasty, thanks to the Habsburgs' ability to produce many offspring and create a multi-branched family tree. Similarly, the War of the Spanish Succession, set into motion by Charles II's death without issue in 1700, marked the end of the Spanish Habsburgs but did not extinguish the dynasty. The Austrian branch, under Emperor Charles

VI, persisted, and his daughter Maria Theresa's accession ensured the dynasty's survival through the Habsburg-Lorraine line. Maria Theresa's reign had much to recommend it; she conquered her enemies and furthered the Habsburgs' ability to adapt to adversity in a time when few women ruled.[129]

The Habsburgs' obstetric outcomes, while not perfect, benefited from their high reproductive output across multiple branches. Maria Theresa's sixteen children, despite some infant mortality, provided an impressive pool of heirs, ensuring that the dynasty could withstand losses that would have crippled a less prolific family. Ferdinand I's fifteen children with Anna of Bohemia and Hungary also generated lots of royal babies, while Philip II's multiple marriages produced many heirs, despite losses. This prolific fertility diluted the impact of inherited genetic mutations, such as Kell incompatibility, which decimated the Tudors' reproductive prospects. The Habsburgs' prodigious fertility all across Europe ensured that no single thing could derail the dynasty, a sharp distinction from the Tudors' reliance on Henry VIII's six marriages, which produced only three surviving legitimate children. The Habsburgs' cultural patronage also played a role in their dynastic success, lending them cachet and prestige across their diverse territories. Rudolf II's court in Prague was an exceptional example of an epicentre of arts and sciences, enhancing the dynasty's cultural reputation. The Spanish Habsburgs, under Philip II, created the Golden Age of Spanish culture, with artists like El Greco and writers like Cervantes basking beneath their royal patronage.[130]

This cultural investment strengthened the dynasty's legitimacy, uniting disparate regions under a shared Habsburg identity. The Tudors, while patrons of Hans Holbein the Younger, who hailed from the Holy Roman Empire, focused more on their own English traditions, with very little emphasis on cultural projection abroad, thus limiting their ability to shape a similar narrative. The Tudors' reproductive strategy, reliant on a single male heir, was fatally undermined by Kell incompatibility and atypical cystic fibrosis, leaving the dynasty with insufficient successors. Elizabeth I's decision not to marry, influenced by the dynasty's troubled reproductive history, sealed its extinction in 1603, marking the end of the Tudor line and the transition to Stuart rule.

The Habsburgs, despite facing similar inbreeding challenges, thrived through a multi-branch structure, prolific reproduction, and brilliant strategic adaptability. Their ability to produce heirs across regions, accept female rulers, when necessary, maintain a vast network of alliances, and utilize economic and cultural resources ensured their survival across the centuries. In contrast, the Tudors' failure to overcome genetic problems and have a more flexible dynastic formula led to their downfall. The Habsburgs' success highlights the power of resilience, foresight, and bountiful offspring, differing from the Tudor dynasty's tragic collapse. The Hapsburg dynasty is a testament to the enduring strength of a well-crafted dynastic plan.

Chapter 4

The Scottish Progeny

The wind rattles the wooden shutters of the stone keep like teeth inside an old woman's head. I close my ears to the sound of it as I sit contemplating the bit of embroidery inside the hoop that lies in my lap. I once lovingly stitched his crest here – the red heart of Douglas – and stupidly I thought his own heart might soften toward me. Now I cannot bear the sight of it. How quickly a man turns his back when his pride is fed by another woman's amorous eyes. The gulls outside cry fierce and hollow, and I envy them. If I had wings I could fly far away from this place – far from false vows and cruel hands. Far, far away from a court that smiles at me in daylight and whispers daggers in the night.

In the waning weeks of 1501, Margaret Beaufort, the stout-hearted matriarch of the Tudor dynasty, stood before her son, Henry VII, and his queen, Elizabeth of York, with an unusual request – to keep their daughter Margaret home for a few more years before marrying her off to a Scottish king much older than herself. She warned them of the dangers this union would have for so young a girl- she could easily be harmed in the marriage bed. Henry VII would not be deterred however, and at the age of just 13, Margaret married James Stuart of Scotland; a union created in order to make peace, but fraught with personal peril for young Margaret. The Treaty of Perpetual Peace, sealed in 1502, dispatched Margaret to Scotland in her thirteenth year, a decision that shaped her life and I believe, her tragic obstetrical history.[131]

Margaret Tudor, the elder sister of Henry VIII, occupies a central place in the Tudor story, and her reproductive struggles echo closely to those of her sisters-in-law, Katherine of Aragon and Anne Boleyn. Across these three women's lives, a troubling pattern emerges: an infant loss rate of around seventy per cent, with spontaneous abortions, stillbirths and the tragic deaths of little babies casting dark shadows over their dynastic aspirations. Margaret was most probably a carrier of the Kell-positive blood group, a rare genetic trait inherited through her mother, Elizabeth of York, which triggered haemolytic disease of the foetus and newborn (HDFN) in her pregnancies, causing many of her infants to be stillborn. Through a meticulous examination of Margaret's obstetrical record, examined with modern genetic insights, with the added comparisons of Katherine and Anne's births, I will attempt an in-depth analysis of Katherine's 'New Year's Prince' and Margaret's son Alexander, both brief-lived infants. I propose a compelling case for the Kell-positive blood group hypothesis, illuminating the genetic mutations that plagued the Tudor and Stuart successions.

Born on 28 November 1489, Margaret Tudor was the first daughter of Henry VII and Elizabeth of York, a union that reconciled the warring houses of Lancaster and York. Henry VII, along with his indomitable mother Margaret Beaufort, were the shrewd architects of Tudor legitimacy. Henry, like most monarchs, viewed his children as diplomatic tools to be used as he saw fit. He arranged their marriages as a means of creating alliances in order to secure his dynasty's fragile claim. Despite Margaret Beaufort's impassioned pleas, the 1502 Treaty of Perpetual Peace betrothed Margaret to James IV of Scotland, a monarch whose charisma and political acumen made him a formidable ally. The marriage was solemnised on 8 August 1503 at Holyrood Palace. The wedding was a lavish affair with young Margaret dressed in a stunning silk gown embroidered with sparkling golden thread. She rode in a gilded carriage drawn by pure white horses, just like a fairytale princess. Jousting competitions and festive masques were held in her honour. The marriage was by proxy with the Earl of Bothwell standing in for the groom. The wedding featured pipers, drummers, and heralds, and was described as marking the beginning of a new era. Yet beneath this pageantry lay an unspoken decree: Margaret's duty would be to produce a male heir, ideally several, to cement the Stuart succession and stabilise Anglo-Scottish relations, a burden that would define her queenship.[132]

As queen consort, Margaret landed in an unfamiliar court where her fertility was her primary currency, her young womb the crucible in which the hopes of two kingdoms would place their futures. Her pregnancies, spanning 1506 to 1514 with James IV, and a final one in 1515 with her second husband, Archibald Douglas, Earl of Angus, were coldly seen as political acts, scrutinised by nobles in Edinburgh and her brother's English court. Of her six pregnancies with James IV, only one child, James V, survived to adulthood, while two daughters were stillborn, and two sons perished in infancy, a nearly seventy per cent mortality rate. This heartbreaking pattern, coupled with the emotional and political consequences of two long standing enemies striving for peace replicates the reproductive challenges faced by queens Katherine of Aragon and Anne Boleyn. Their loss rates were also 70 per cent, suggesting a shared genetic thread - the Kell-positive blood group, woven through the Tudor lineage.

Unlike Owen Tudor, James Stuart had the decency to wait a couple of years before consummating his marriage with young Margaret Tudor, allowing her to finish growing and maturing both emotionally and physically. Her obstetrical journey began in the autumn of 1506, at the age of 16, when she conceived her first child, a moment of promise for the Stuart-Tudor alliance. On 21 February 1507, she gave birth to James, Prince of Scotland, at Holyrood Palace, an event met with jubilation across the realm. No expense was spared on the baby's household, including an ornate cradle of oak draped in crimson velvet, swaddling clothes of fine Holland cloth, and a silver christening font commissioned from Edinburgh goldsmiths. There were celebrations amongst the Scots and at court, with James IV hosting banquets and tournaments to honour his new princeling. Sadly, the Scottish kingdom's moment of triumph was fleeting; baby James died in February 1508 at Stirling Castle, aged 1 year. In a letter from James IV to Henry VII, the Scottish king expressed sorrow and disappointment but resolved to try again. This loss, which occurred as Margaret was already pregnant with her second child, initiated a relentless cycle of hope and despair, which would echo that of her sister-in-law Katherine of Aragon.

In July 1508, Margaret gave birth for the second time, to an unnamed daughter at Holyrood; sadly, the baby was either stillborn or dead within hours, a tragedy recorded with stark brevity: 'The queen was delivered of a daughter, but it lived not'. Margaret was devastated. James IV presented a magnificent sapphire ring to Margaret, presumably a gift to console her during her grief. This second loss, following so closely on the first, deepened young Margaret's private sorrow, though her public role demanded stoic endurance in a court that expected another heir post haste.[133]

Margaret's third pregnancy, conceived in early 1509, brought renewed hope for the kingdom. On 20 October 1509, she gave birth to Arthur, Prince of Scotland, at Holyrood Palace. The baby was named Arthur, evoking the king of the Arthurian legends and Margaret's late brother, Prince Arthur. This was a deliberate tribute to her Tudor heritage, demonstrating her intent to strengthen her familial and dynastic ties. There were jubilant celebrations at court, with James IV ordering a tournament in honour of the occasion. Yet baby Arthur's health faltered, and he too perished on 14 July 1510 at Edinburgh Castle, aged nine months old, another big blow for the dynasty. James sent a letter to Henry VIII, noting the death with diplomatic restraint. Margaret's grief, compounded by the rapid succession of pregnancies and losses, crushed her resilience, again duplicating the physical and emotional tolls Katherine of Aragon would endure.[134]

On 10 April 1512, Margaret gave birth to James V at Linlithgow Palace, a baby boy who was destined to survive and ascend the Scottish throne, securing the Stuart line. King James sent a proud proclamation to Henry VIII, writing of his heir's good health. A grand christening was held, featuring a beautiful silver-gilt font, velvet canopies embroidered with gold, and a choir of fifty singers. The baby's birth was a triumph, with bonfires lit across Edinburgh in celebration. This success, however, was overshadowed by another loss in late 1512 or early 1513, when Margaret delivered another unnamed daughter, probably stillborn.[135]

'The queen was brought to bed of a daughter, but it was not viable.' The lack of any recorded expenses for a christening or household suggests that the baby's birth was a tragedy that passed unrecorded in the court's bustle. Surely the death of another daughter had a grim impact on Margaret's emotional state, and the constant childbearing would have had a deleterious effect on her physical health.

Unfortunately, things were about to take a profound turn for the worse for Margaret. The premature death of Margaret's husband James IV at the Battle of Flodden, on 9 September 1513, (orchestrated by none other than Queen Regent Katherine of Aragon), thrust Margaret into the role of regent for her infant son James V. This position was fraught with political peril amidst a court divided by factionalism and suspicious of a woman in a powerful role. Margaret's sixth pregnancy, conceived before Flodden, culminated on 24 April 1514 with the birth of Alexander, Duke of Ross, at Stirling Castle. The country held its collective breath to see if this tiny heir would survive, with Margaret herself presiding over the baptism ceremony despite her queenship burdens. Tragically, Alexander died on 18 December 1515, aged twenty months and Margaret lamented in a letter to her brother Henry VIII that she suspected foul play by the Duke of Albany, though no evidence supports this claim. Her anguish, compounded by political intrigue, reveals the depths of her loss, set against the backdrop of a kingdom in great upheaval.[136]

In 1514, Margaret married again to Archibald Douglas, a controversial union frowned upon by rivalling nobility. Margaret lost the regency to her son to John Stuart, Duke of Albany. In 1515, pregnant by her second husband, Margaret fled to England amidst dangerous political turmoil. On 8 October 1515, she gave birth to Margaret Douglas at Harbottle Castle, a beautiful daughter who survived to become Countess of Lennox and mother of Henry Stuart, Lord Darnley. Margaret remained in exile after the birth of her baby daughter, and a letter from Margaret to Henry VIII described the birth amidst terrible hardship. Little Margaret's christening cost a trifling £200, quite a contrast to her siblings' grand Scottish ceremonies.[137] This rare reproductive success stood in sharp relief against the losses with James IV, suggesting a different genetic dynamic with Douglas.

Margaret's obstetrical record with James IV – six pregnancies, two likely stillborn daughters (1508, 1512–1513), two infant deaths (1507, 1509), and one surviving son (1512) – presents a nearly 70 per cent loss rate, corresponding with the seventy per cent loss rates of Katherine and Anne. The pattern of initial success followed by escalating losses, marked by stillbirths and early deaths, paints us the picture of a serious medical problem, probably haemolytic disease of the newborn, caused by Kell-positive blood group incompatibility, possibly worsened by the early reproductive demands placed on a 15-year-old girl, which Margaret Beaufort had tried to warn Henry Vll about.

The Kell antigen, a rare blood group trait present in approximately nine per cent of populations, can trigger haemolytic disease of the newborn when a Kell-negative mother develops potent anti-K antibodies after exposure to a Kell-positive foetus, typically during her first pregnancy. These antibodies attack the red blood cells of subsequent Kell-positive babies in utero, causing severe anaemia that leads to miscarriages, stillbirths, or neonatal deaths. Unlike Rh incompatibility, Kell-related haemolytic disease of the newborn is more severe, with antibodies capable of causing children in the womb to perish as early as the second trimester. The hallmark of Kell-induced haemolytic disease is an initial successful pregnancy followed by increasing losses of future children, a pattern that aligns strikingly with Margaret's obstetrical history, making the Kell-positive hypothesis the most logical explanation for her stillbirths.

For Margaret to have been a Kell-positive carrier, she would have inherited the K allele, which researchers have traced back to her maternal great grandmother Jacquetta of Luxembourg (see Part 2, Chapter 1). If James IV was Kell-positive or a carrier, their babies had a high probability of being Kell-positive, triggering haemolytic disease of the newborn in a Kell-negative Margaret or, conversely, in a Kell-positive Margaret paired with a Kell-negative husband. The survival of Margaret Douglas with Archibald Douglas in 1515 suggests good genetic compatibility possibly because Douglas was Kell-negative, reducing the risk of haemolytic disease of the newborn. This genetic drama, though unprovable without modern forensic testing, provides a framework for understanding Margaret's losses. The early pregnancies, beginning at age 15 after her marriage at 13, may have exacerbated the physical toll, potentially weakening Margaret's capacity to sustain healthy pregnancies and amplifying the impact of genetic incompatibilities.

Margaret's obstetrical history reveals a haunting pattern suggesting Kell-induced haemolytic disease of the newborn. Her first pregnancy in 1507 produced James, who survived for just one year, suggesting initial compatibility or a lack of significant antibody response. Baby James' death in 1508, possibly from natural causes or mild haemolytic disease with complications like neonatal anaemia, marked the beginning of a string of Margaret's losses. The stillbirth of a daughter in July 1508, could represent a 'sensitizing' event, where a Kell-negative mother (Margaret in this case) developed anti-K antibodies against a Kell-positive foetus during a later pregnancy. This rapid loss, with no recorded christening or household expenses, underscores the physical and emotional trauma experienced by a young teenaged queen recovering from her first labour.

The birth of Arthur in October 1509, followed by his tragic death at just nine months in July 1510, could imply mild haemolytic effects, with postnatal complications such as anaemia or jaundice contributing to his death. The queen held out hope along with her court of the little boy's survival, yet the historical records note his death with shocking brevity, offering no cause at all, or even speculation as to the circumstances of his death. The survival of James V, born in April 1512, demonstrates that he must have been Kell-negative, meaning that he successfully evaded his mother's antibodies, or it's also possible that Margaret's antibody levels were temporarily reduced. The stillbirth of a daughter in late 1512 or early 1513 demonstrates the signs typically seen in severe haemolytic disease. This loss of yet another child further increased Margaret's cataclysmic distress during the political fallout of James IV's impending campaign against England. It's hard to imagine a more devastating situation for Margaret than having to deliver a dead child during such a politically fraught period.

Alexander's birth in April 1514, during Margaret's precarious regency, and his death in December 1515, is interesting. It may reflect postnatal haemolytic disease complications, such as jaundice or organ failure, although his twenty-month survival suggests other factors were at play, maybe illness or malnutrition, which could have slid under the radar during the regency's chaos. However, Margaret had a suspicion, which she reports to her brother Henry VIII, of foul play, but it is unsupported by evidence. It's possible to imagine that her suspicions were the result of extreme emotional distress in combination with the politically fraught situation.[138]

The survival of baby daughter Margaret Douglas in October 1515, a child fathered by Archibald Douglas during exile, is pivotal. Margaret had to contend with her pregnancy amidst her flight to England in what must have been an incredibly stressful period for her. The successful birth and survival of Margaret Douglas proves that she did not contribute a Kell-positive allele, or Margaret's antibodies did not affect this baby, reducing the haemolytic disease risk.*

* I do find it fascinating and worthy of note that out of the three queens who suffered from this genetic disorder, all of the surviving children of these women were female. I do not have a plausible explanation for this phenomenon, but I do think it is extraordinary.

The contrast with her losses with James IV – two stillbirths and two infant deaths – strengthens the Kell hypothesis, as paternal genetics are critical in haemolytic disease of the newborn.

Margaret's high neonatal loss rate perfectly aligns with modern estimates of untreated Kell-related haemolytic disease rates, which can cause fifty to eighty per cent foetal or neonatal loss. Contemporary sources of Margaret Tudor's time can provide no explanations, reflecting the era's utter lack of understanding of blood group incompatibilities. The sequential pattern – initial success followed by escalating losses – offers compelling evidence that Margaret was a Kell-positive carrier, her stillbirths a tragic consequence of genetic blood group incompatibility, worsened by the early reproductive demands on her immature young body.

The tragedy of Margaret's losses finds a striking parallel in the short life of Katherine of Aragon and Henry VIII's 'New Year's Prince', Henry, Duke of Cornwall, born on 1 January 1511 and dead by 22 February 1511, aged seven weeks. King Henry was elated and ordered lavish celebrations at Richmond Palace, with £2000 spent on tournaments, feasts, and pageants, including a masque where Henry VIII played a golden knight. He sent out birth announcements to European courts proclaiming the Tudor prince. Yet the prince's sudden death, with no cause specified, thrust the court into mourning, with Katherine's grief captured in a Letters and Papers entry: 'The queen weeps daily for her lost son'.[139]

Margaret's son, Alexander, Duke of Ross, born on 24 April 1514 at Stirling Castle and dead by 18 December 1515, aged twenty months, shares similarities with the New Year's Prince, raising the question of whether both succumbed to haemolytic disease of the newborn caused by Kell-positive blood group incompatibility. Alexander's christening was attended by Scottish nobles and was celebrated with crimson banners and an elaborate silver font for the baptism. Contemporary sources note the hope invested in this second son, with Margaret presiding despite regency pressures. Her letter to Henry VIII laments his loss, suspecting foul play by Albany, though no biological cause is mentioned, typical of the era's records.

There are striking similarities between Katherine and Margaret's baby boys who survived birth but died early, indicating postnatal vulnerability distinct from Margaret's stillborn daughters. The New

Year's Prince's seven-week survival suggests mild haemolytic disease, where a Kell-positive foetus, born to a Kell-negative mother – in this case Katherine – succumbed to complications like jaundice or anaemia, as maternal antibodies attacked his red blood cells. Alexander's twenty-month survival could point to a similarly mild haemolytic disease effect, with postnatal anaemia contributing, though his longer life suggests additional factors, such as illness during Margaret's turbulent regency. Both losses align with haemolytic disease of the newborn, with a pattern of escalating in severity after a sensitising pregnancy, with Margaret's multiple losses (1507–1513) and Katherine's prior miscarriage in 1510 indicating antibody accumulation. If Henry VIII and Margaret, siblings sharing Elizabeth of York's lineage, were Kell-positive, their Kell-positive foetuses faced haemolytic disease risks with Kell-negative partners (Katherine, James IV), tying these infants' fates to a shared genetic legacy.

The New Year's Prince's shorter survival (seven weeks) versus Alexander's twenty months suggests differences in haemolytic disease severity or external factors. The New Year's Prince's death, early in Katherine's reproductive history, may reflect a milder antibody response, as her 1510 miscarriage was her first sensitising event. Alexander's death, following Margaret's five prior pregnancies, certainly indicates a stronger antibody response, yet his longer survival suggests milder haemolytic disease or even environmental factors, like contagion or neglect during Scotland's political instability. The New Year's Prince's death took place in a stable English court, while Alexander's death happened during Scotland's chaos, highlighting contextual differences. The New Year's Prince's christening was a much more lavish affair, reflecting England's wealth and stability, but both ceremonies masked the infants' fragility.

Margaret's probable Kell-positive status may have originated with Elizabeth of York, whose reproductive history offers clues to her carrier status. Elizabeth, daughter of Edward IV and Elizabeth Woodville, had seven pregnancies with two infant deaths, yielding a twenty-nine per cent loss rate. While this is lower than Margaret's or Katherine's rates, this suggests Elizabeth probably carried the K allele, passed to Margaret and Henry VIII. The marriage of Elizabeth to Henry VII, uniting York and Lancaster, concentrated the Tudor gene pool, amplifying rare alleles like Kell. This dynastic merger produced siblings whose reproductive challenges suggest a shared hereditary factor.

The absence of close consanguinity in Margaret's marriage to James IV – they were fourth cousins once removed – rules out inbreeding, which reinforces the hypothesis of a Tudor-specific trait. Elizabeth Woodville's ten children with Edward IV, with few recorded losses, suggest the K allele entered through Elizabeth of York's paternal line, probably through Jacquetta of Luxembourg. This offers no genetic insights, but the pattern across Elizabeth's children – Margaret's stillbirths, Henry's losses with Katherine and Anne – points us to a shared Kell-positive legacy.

Margaret's losses exacted a profound emotional toll, binding her to Katherine and Anne Boleyn in shared sorrow. A 1515 letter, written from exile, reveals her despair over Alexander's death and her lost regency, her words heavy with grief: 'My heart is sore for my son, and my crown is lost'.[140] The poignant letter describes her relentless pregnancies, six in eight years, and her loss of agency, mirroring the experiences of Katherine and Anne. These relentless pregnancies amplified Kell risks, as each pregnancy increased antibody exposure, turning hope into heartbreak.

Politically, Margaret's seventy per cent loss rate weakened her regency post-Flodden. Then there were her struggles against Albany, with James V's survival anchoring the Stuart line. Her 1514 marriage to Archibald Douglas, a unity made to secure political allies, cost her her regency, as nobles questioned her loyalty. Katherine's loss of so many babies fanned the flames of Henry's doubts, leading to the annulment. Anne's losses, including a 1536 stillbirth, precipitated her execution, in a letter written by Ambassador Chapuys to Charles V, he states 'Anne has miscarried of her savior'. These tragedies transformed private grief into dynastic catastrophes.

Emotionally, Margaret's grief, Katherine's sorrow, and Anne's despair reflect shared emotional burdens under public scrutiny. Margaret's resilience, seen in Margaret Douglas's survival, parallels Katherine's legacy through Mary and Anne's through Elizabeth, defying a genetic curse.

Margaret Tudor's role as queen consort of Scotland extended far beyond her personal tragedies, positioning her as a linchpin in the delicate balance of Anglo-Scottish relations during a period of volatile diplomacy. The Treaty of Perpetual Peace, sealed in 1502 was not merely a marriage contract but also a bold attempt to end centuries of border conflicts, with Margaret's fertility as its trump card. Her reproductive outcomes, scrutinised in both Edinburgh and London, carried profound implications for the Tudor-Stuart alliance, shaping the trajectory of two kingdoms and the eventual union of their crowns. Margaret's obstetrical challenges had a profound impact on the Anglo-Scottish diplomacy and affected the course of the Stuart legacy. The history reveals intense diplomatic activity surrounding Margaret's arrival in Scotland in 1503, with Henry VII dispatching envoys to ensure her welcome, reflecting the treaty's gravitas. The accounts of the Lord High Treasurer of Scotland record £2000 spent on her coronation, an enormous sum of money for that time rivalling James IV's annual revenue, showing Scotland's commitment to the alliance. However, the treaty's success hinged on Margaret producing a male heir to unite the Stuart and Tudor bloodlines, a pressure evident in James IV's letters to Henry VIII, urging patience as Margaret matured into motherhood. Scottish enthusiasm for the Anglo alliance from nobles like the Earl of Huntly was evident in the festivities and feasts in honour of Margaret's potential to secure the succession. This expectation placed Margaret under tremendous pressure, her body treated like a diplomatic asset whose failures risked unravelling the fragile alliance of two important kingdoms.

The early loss of Margaret's children, while deeply personal, reverberated through Anglo-Scottish relations. A 1508 letter from Henry VIII to James IV, expressing condolence for the death of Margaret's first son but urging continued alliance, was a reminder that dynastic hopes outweighed personal grief. Henry VIII's underlying concern was that Margaret's losses could embolden Scottish nobles to question the treaty's value, prompting him to send £500 in gifts to boost up Margaret's standing.[141] By 1510, after the death of her son Arthur, murmurs among the Scottish council grew, with some members advocating for James IV to seek a new alliance with France, that perennial thorn in the side of England. Margaret's inability to produce a surviving heir until 1512 strained the treaty, as both courts deeply feared a succession crisis that could reignite border wars, a fear compounded by Henry VIII's ascension in 1509 and his aggressive stance against Scotland.[142]

The birth of James V in 1512, was celebrated with £1500 in christening expenses, and reinvigorated the alliance, with Henry VIII holding feasts at his English court in celebration of his nephew. James V's christening was a rite with diplomatic opportunities, with both French and Danish envoys clinking glasses, highlighting Scotland's strengthened position. The tragic loss of a daughter in 1513 coincided with James IV's fatal

Flodden campaign and plunged the Anglo/Scottish alliance into a crisis. Henry VIII's letter to Margaret offered support for her regency but he also demanded that her primary loyalty be to England, a demand that complicated her precarious position as a Tudor in a grieving Scottish court. Margaret's regency was seriously weakened by her losses, and it became something of a diplomatic tightrope, with the Duke of Albany's correspondence revealing his intent to align Scotland with France, undermining the Tudor-Stuart bond.[143]

Margaret's exile in 1515 and the birth of Margaret Douglas at Harbottle Castle, marked by an extremely modest christening, demonstrates a turning point. Henry VIII's letter was an avuncular welcoming for baby Margaret, but his refusal to intervene in Scotland, citing financial strain, reflects the alliance's tenuous position. Margaret Douglas's survival became a major diplomatic asset. Her marriage to Matthew Stuart, Earl of Lennox, was arranged by her uncle Henry VIII, thereby reinforcing diplomatic ties between England and Scotland. The role of Margaret Douglas in the Stuart lineage became an important lynchpin after her son Henry Stuart, Lord Darnley married Mary, Queen of Scots. This union paved the way for James VI's claim to the English throne in 1603. James V's survival, meanwhile, ensured the Stuart succession, with his daughter Mary's birth in 1542 further linking together the two dynasties. Margaret's children, despite her many losses, fulfilled the goal of the Treaty of Perpetual Peace's vision in its unity of the Scottish and English crowns a century later.

Comparatively, Spanish Infanta Katherine of Aragon's role as the Queen Consort informed England's foreign policy. Her marriage to Henry VIII in 1509 secured an important and powerful Spanish alliance against France. Katherine's heartbreaking failure to produce a surviving male heir, beyond the New Year's Prince, strained this alliance and weakened England's dynastic stability. Katherine's diplomatic efforts, hosting Spanish envoys and advocating for her daughter Mary's rights, parallel Margaret's regency struggles. These women leveraged their natal ties to bolster their positions. Anne Boleyn's brief tenure as queen consort shifted England toward Protestant alliances, with her unfortunate losses prompting Henry VIII to seek French support. Anne's failure to produce a male heir, like Margaret's and Katherine's, destabilised England's foreign policy, echoing Margaret's impact on Anglo/Scottish relations.

Chapter 5

Ephemeral Progeny

A tiny court of golden-haired children laugh and dance before me, their sweet voices somehow familiar to me, as if I had known them before. Perhaps I have, perhaps these little ones were my lost brothers and sisters – or they are the children God had ordained for me to bring into this world. But I was not worthy. I have lost Callais and I have lost Phillip, and I never had the chance to meet the children of my body, for now I must be gone from this world and my crown will sit upon another's head. The one that is daughter to that black eyed witch who cast out my mother and seduced my father. My babies call to me! I'm coming, I say to them. Wait for me...

1516 was an excellent year for the royal house of Tudor. On February 18, Queen Katherine of Aragon gave birth to a healthy baby girl. Although this was not the prince King Henry craved, he was nonetheless delighted to have a thriving child in the nursery after so many losses. Princess Mary was the apple of her father's eye and adored by her mother who had years of pent-up maternal urgings with no live baby to fulfil them with. Mary's birth was a triumph, though not the son Henry desired. 'We are young yet, and God willing sons will follow', Henry said to his wife with a smile that belied his deeper hopes.

Greenwich Palace was nestled along the Thames River with beautiful sprawling gardens and luxurious tapestried rooms – it housed the Tudor court at the time of Mary's birth. The courtiers along with the whole of England celebrated with feasts, music, and great good cheer. Mary's christening was a grand affair, attended by nobles, clergy, and dignitaries; it is believed that Queen Katherine chose her name to honour the Virgin Mary, reflecting Katherine's deep love of Catholicism. Ambassadors from France, Spain, and the Holy Roman Empire attended the christening, no doubt pondering future betrothals for the princess that could bind England to Europe's greater powers. A healthy, legitimate princess was a valuable diplomatic asset for England.[144]

Katherine flouted royal custom by keeping Mary close, overseeing her care with fierce devotion. The nursery at Greenwich was a sanctuary of warmth and routine, and filled with the soft voices of the baby's household. Margaret Pole, Countess of Salisbury was given the position of governess, just as she had once cared for the king and his sisters. Additionally, she shared her monarchs' Catholic piety which made her an ideal governess for the little princess. Margaret was a descendant of the House of York, and she brought loyalty and experience to her role, ensuring that Mary's early years were full of lessons that were appropriate for a princess. Princess Mary thrived and as a copper-haired, blue-eyed child, she was a true daughter of the house of Tudor. She was remarkably intelligent and gifted in many areas. Her rosy cheeks and alert gaze charmed the court, evoking praise from all and sundry.[145]

The Tudor court of 1516 was a vibrant stage for Henry's youthful charisma. Only 24 at the time of Mary's birth, Henry was ascending to his prime while his wife had begun to lose her girlish looks and was worn out from repeated childbearing. The absence of a male heir cast a deepening shadow, growing with each passing year. Mary's birth offered a brief respite, but Katherine was still under immense pressure to produce a son. Courtiers, from ambitious nobles to foreign envoys, saw in the princess a new, shiny piece in the diplomatic puzzle, her future marriage a potential bridge to France, Spain, or the Holy Roman Empire.

Katherine poured her maternal heart into Mary's upbringing, determined to raise a princess as learned as any prince. By the age of 3, Mary was already starting to read, her lisping voice repeating Latin prayers under her mother's watchful eye. Katherine, with a humanist education, believed princesses needed skills for court and diplomatic challenges. She hired tutors to teach Mary music and dancing, as well as Greek and Latin, but religion remained the primary focus of her education. The queen's piety was as much a part of her as her crown; she taught Mary Catholic devotion with Mary's rosary beads becoming a constant companion in her small hands. These early lessons shaped a little girl who was both bright and impressionable, her natural intelligence always remarked upon by those who met her. 'Her mind is beyond her years', one tutor remarked, a sentiment echoed by courtiers who saw in her the makings of a formidable royal.[146]

Henry's affection for his daughter was genuine, though tempered by the pressures of kingship. In 1518, when Mary was 2, he presented her at a banquet for French ambassadors during negotiations for the Treaty of London, a short-lived plan for European peace. Lifting her high, he called her 'my pearl', and the guests marvelled at the pretty, precocious toddler. The French envoys, charmed by the adorable child, noted her potential as a future bride, though such talks were perhaps premature. Henry's pride was evident, but his deeper concern over the lack of a male heir never faded. A daughter could forge alliances through marriage, but only a son could ensure the Tudor throne's unbroken line.[147]

Mary's early childhood was a balance of royal splendour and strict routine. She travelled with her parents to palaces like Richmond, Windsor, and Eltham, carried through halls adorned with gold-threaded tapestries and elaborate chandeliers. At Eltham Palace, where she spent much of her time, Mary was an apt pupil for the lessons taught to her by her tutors. These rigorous lessons contrasted sharply with the court's adoration of glamour where every event was a carefully orchestrated display of conspicuous consumption. Katherine made sure that Mary's household was staffed with loyal servants who shared her rigorous Catholic values, creating a well sheltered environment for the princess. Margaret Pole remained a constant presence, guiding Mary with a blend of discipline and affection.[148]

Mary's daily life at Eltham followed a structured rhythm that reflected Katherine's meticulous care. Mornings focused on reading, writing, basic Latin grammar, and simple prayers with tutors. Afternoons brought music practice or needlework, skills deemed essential for all princesses. Mary took to the virginals early, playing melodies that impressed courtiers and attendants. Mary's evenings ended with prayers with Katherine usually joining her daughter and overseeing her bedtime routine. The queen also introduced Mary to Spanish literature, reading to her daughter tales of saints' lives to inspire her with greater faith.

By 1520, when Mary was 4, her role in diplomacy began to take shape. The Field of the Cloth of Gold, an opulent diplomatic meeting between

Henry and King Francis I of France, served as an occasion to propose Mary as a possible candidate for marriage to the French dauphin. The negotiations failed, but highlighted Mary's increasing worth in Europe's marriage market. In 1522, at the age of 6, Mary became the centrepiece of a significant diplomatic triumph: she became engaged to her cousin, Charles V, Holy Roman Emperor, and king of Spain. Formalised through the Treaty of Bruges, the engagement bound England to the most powerful ruler in Europe, Katherine's nephew, whose vast empire spanned Spain, the Netherlands, parts of Italy, and the New World. For Henry, this alliance represented a calculated strategy to offset the growing influence of France within Europe. For Katherine, it was a very personal victory that tied her daughter to her beloved Spain and ensured Mary's future as a queen of unparalleled influence. Henry thought that this betrothal would become the cornerstone of a Tudor-Habsburg unity, forming strong support against common enemies and propping up the Catholic cause across Europe.[149]

The negotiations began in 1521, when Charles visited England, hosted by Henry in a dazzling display of mutual ambition. Both young rulers viewed the match as a way to strengthen their alliance. At Greenwich, 5-year-old Mary was introduced to Charles, wearing velvet and pearls. The emperor gave her a formal bow and noted her composed demeanour.[150] Gossip at court exploded – this was the most thrilling event to have happened in years. This betrothal was a guarantee of England's proper place at the heart of European power. The terms of the betrothal were intricate, reflecting the delicate balance of diplomacy. Mary was to wed Charles when she reached 12, in 1528, with provisions for her to join his court earlier if it was deemed necessary. Charles pledged critical military support against France while Henry's advisors negotiated a substantial dowry for their monarch's only daughter.[151] To prepare her for her future role, Katherine intensified Mary's education, teaching her Castilian court customs as well as traditional Spanish songs and dances, such as the pavane, to familiarise her with her future husband's culture.[152]

At court, Mary was a much-admired child and a future Empress; as such she was treated with deferential respect. Her lessons were adjusted to focus on the diplomatic skills required for Charles's cosmopolitan court. Yet the bridegroom himself remained a distant figure, his letters to Mary were formal and infrequent as he juggled wars and political crises across his empire. By 1525, however, cracks in the betrothal began to appear. Charles was under considerable pressure from his advisors due to financial strains from his far-flung empire and so became hesitant about the marriage. The sixteen-year age difference, combined with his need for a rich bride who could produce heirs immediately, led him to decide against the match with Mary. In 1527, he broke the engagement and decided instead to marry the wealthy Isabella of Portugal, a decision that stung Katherine deeply and humiliated Henry on the European stage. For Mary, still a very small girl, the dissolution was probably disappointing, but she was much too young to appreciate the impact this had on her parents. Katherine, disappointed but undeterred, continued to prepare her daughter for a grand future, teaching her to see such setbacks as tests of faith and resilience.[153]

Mary's humanist education continued with the best tutors to be found in England. At the tender age of 6, she studied Latin and French with a rigour rare for a girl of her age, her tutors, including the scholar John Veysey, later Bishop of Exeter, praising her sharp mind. Music became a particular passion; Mary's skill on the virginals drew admiration at court events, where she performed with a poise that belied her years. Her musical flair was a point of pride for her father who was a masterful musician himself, and his daughter Mary's prodigy was worthy of the crown. Katherine ensured that Mary's studies balanced her studies with Catholic doctrines, drawing on the lives of saintly women like Catherine of Siena to inspire her daughter's faith. Mary's fluency in Latin grew to such levels that she was able to correspond with scholars, a skill that impressed even the most sceptical courtiers and reinforced her role as a royal prodigy.

The broader court, meanwhile, was growing tense. Katherine's pregnancies had ceased by the early 1520s, and Henry's frustration over the lack of a male heir fuelled gossip of dynastic instability. The king's affections were drawn to younger ladies-in-waiting at court, notably Anne Boleyn, whose sharp wit and French *savoir faire* contrasted with Katherine's quiet dignity. Mary, still a child, remained oblivious to these courtly undercurrents, shielded by her governess Margaret Pole. Katherine fortified Mary's household with trusted nurses, tutors, and chaplains devoted to the queen's Catholic beliefs so that her daughter's inner circle remained far from unsavoury influences.[154]

In 1525, when Mary was 9, Henry made a bold and unprecedented decision: he named her Princess of Wales, a title traditionally reserved for the male inheritor of the throne. It was a bold move, signalling his acceptance of Mary as his heir despite her sex. Mary was sent to Ludlow Castle in the Welsh Marches to preside over the Council of the Marches, a role that introduced her to the responsibilities of governance. Accompanied by Margaret Pole and a retinue of trusted advisors, she lived apart from her parents in her own household in the rugged Welsh countryside.

Life at Ludlow was a microcosm of the royal court, with its own rhythms and rituals. Mary's household included young nobles like Jane Dormer, who later became a close confidante, and priests who reinforced her Catholic upbringing. Her routine included administrative tasks, teaching, devotions, and riding with her master-of-horse and pony. Mary became an accomplished rider at Ludlow, exploring the castle grounds and nearby areas. She practised new music or read letters from her parents and worked on her embroidery. Mary corresponded with her father in beautifully inked Latin; her letters filled with formal respect and words of daughterly affection.[155]

Court pageantry remained a constant in Mary's life, even from afar. At Christmas 1524, before her departure to Ludlow, she joined her parents at Greenwich for a celebration marked by masques, feasts, and music. Dressed magnificently in velvet and jewels, she danced with young nobles, her steps graceful and precise from hours of practice. These events, carefully orchestrated, reinforced the Tudor dynasty's projection of opulence, with Mary's presence one of the most elements. But beneath the splendour, trouble was brewing in Henry and Katherine's marriage. Henry, it was gossiped, was considering putting his loyal wife aside in hopes of a younger and more fertile wife. It would become an emotionally fraught period for Mary who would come to suffer terribly due to her father's duplicity towards her mother.[156]

Mary's early years shimmered with promise as she basked in her parents' love and the Tudor court's approval. In 1526, at the age of 10, she was still residing at Ludlow Castle, presiding over a court that affirmed her royal status. However, Henry, desperate for a male heir, began questioning his marriage to Katherine. Henry cited Leviticus as his way of arguing that the marriage between him and his brother's former wife was cursed for lack of sons. For young Mary, this was not mere politics but a personal unravelling. Her parents' estrangement rocked her secure world, plunging her deep into emotional torment. At the age of 12 in 1528, Mary's anxiety continued to deepen. When she was sent back to court amidst the annulment debates, she witnessed her mother's defiance and the king's growing affection for Anne Boleyn. The Spanish ambassador, Eustace Chapuys, was a stalwart defender of Queen Katherine; he reported Mary's 'sorrow' and 'weakness' as she grappled with her mother's precarious position. Mary's health faltered, with 'pains in her stomach' and irregular menstruation, early signs of endometrial damage. These symptoms, described as 'The Mother' or 'suffocation of the matrix', at the time, reflected the Tudor physicians' vague understanding of gynaecological issues.[157] There was deep turmoil for the princess as Mary's world transformed from one of love, admiration and high status to something else entirely. The annulment dragged on, with papal delays fuelling Henry's impatience. The imminent dissolution of her parents' marriage, and the fallout from this estrangement would cause tremendous grief and fear that would permanently scar Mary's psyche. Mary's chronic emotional distress during these formative years served to disrupt her endocrine system and impact her health in profound ways. Psychological trauma would soon manifest itself in excruciatingly painful menstrual cycles as Mary began to mature into a young woman.

The years 1531 to 1533, ages 15 to 17, marked the apex of Mary's suffering. In 1531, Henry banished Katherine from court, severing Mary's contact with her mother, who was confined to Kimbolton Castle. A letter from Katherine's household describes Mary's 'frequent crying' and pleas to visit her mother, denied by royal decree. This separation was a wound that never healed; Katherine died in 1536, and Mary never saw her again. In 1533, Henry married Anne Boleyn, and declared his marriage to Katherine void, stripping Mary of her title, proclaiming her illegitimate.[158] Spanish Envoy Chapuys cried in outrage: 'The Princess is cast down, her title stolen, her heart broken'.[159] Mary was relegated to the household of her newly born half-sister Elizabeth, daughter of Queen Anne, where she endured the humiliation of becoming a servant to the tiny infant. Mary struggled with 'grief and despair' and 'fear for her life' as she resisted the pressure to accept her demotion. Mary, during these years experienced great sorrow for her lost mother and the increasing court pressures on her to accept Anne as queen. Her emotional turmoil compounded by her father's rejection, loss of status, religious persecution, and social isolation created a state of chronic stress. Chapuys' dispatches described her 'melancholy' and physical weakness, suggesting a young woman buckling under relentless trauma. This psychological burden, as modern science reveals, had profound physiological consequences, particularly on her endocrine system.

The sixteenth century lacked the language to explain the connection to the mind and body, but Mary's suffering is a prime example of how emotional distress can disrupt the body's hormones. Chronic stress like Mary experienced, activates the HPA axis which instructs the body to release cortisol in response to threats. This powerful hormone is useful in the short term, but cortisol in the blood over long periods disrupts the hypothalamic-pituitary-ovarian (HPO) axis, which controls reproductive hormones like oestrogen, progesterone, luteinizing hormone (LH), and follicle-stimulating hormone (FSH). This disruption is bad for a woman's body and can lead to irregular ovulation, painful menstruation, and gynaecological disorders.[160] Mary's adolescent trauma – her grief over her mother's banishment and death, fear of her father's wrath, and isolation in Elizabeth's household, caused Mary so much stress it raised her cortisol levels and prevented the HPO axis from normal functioning. Her 'great sorrow' and 'despair', as Chapuys and court letters describe, paint a picture of a girl in a state of chronic stress. Research has shown that prolonged cortisol exposure will disturb proper ovarian function, contributing to conditions such as endometriosis. While polycystic ovarian syndrome could be the culprit, Mary's symptoms do not match-up well with this diagnosis. Extremely painful periods such as she experienced suggest endometriosis as the cause of her menstrual woes. This diagnosis will fit into a later syndrome as we will explore soon.

Endometriosis is a condition where endometrial tissue grows outside the uterus. It is a condition which causes women to have severe pelvic pain, irregular periods, and infertility; it affects 10–15 per cent of women and it is linked to stress-induced inflammation and hormonal imbalances.[161] Mary's symptoms, documented in contemporary sources, perfectly match this condition, and her adolescent trauma triggered its onset or exacerbation.

From her mid-teens, Mary suffered 'pains in her stomach' and 'The Mother', sixteenth-century terms for severe menstrual pain. Chapuys wrote about her 'disorders of her courses', a reference to irregular menstrual cycles that caused her terrible suffering as well as disruption of her duties. These symptoms also probably included dysmenorrhea, or cessation of menstrual cycles, another symptom of endometriosis. Her distress was severe enough to draw court attention; it must have been a very debilitating condition beyond typical menstrual cramps. Elevated cortisol levels in her blood from her 'grief' and 'fear' disrupted the oestrogen-progesterone balance, causing abnormal endometrial growth in her uterus.[162] The Tudor court's medical interventions of purging and bleeding would have only exacerbated Mary's condition, as they failed to address the root problem.

From 1533, at age 17, when her father, Henry VIII, declared her illegitimate, Mary faced a life of continuous emotional turmoil, religious strife, and political isolation. Her emotional scars that were created in childhood by her parents' divorce and her mother's banishment, deepened, while her fragile health, which was destroyed by chronic gynaecological ailments, continued to grow worse.

Mary's isolation intensified until Anne Boleyn's execution in May 1536, when Mary was 20. Henry's third wife, Jane Seymour, urged Henry to reconcile with his once-beloved daughter Mary. At this point Mary had submitted to her father's supremacy, signing a document acknowledging her illegitimate status and the annulment of her mother's marriage. Thanks to Jane's kindness, Mary found some comfort and received a home at Hunsdon, although her position remained unclear.[163] Even though Mary returned to her father's court, her sadness remained. Her health was fragile, the court physicians attempted to treat her 'weakness' and 'disorders of her courses', no doubt bleeding her and making her even more unwell.

Jane's death in 1537, after giving birth to Edward, meant more queen stepmothers to contend with. Mary served as a lady-in-waiting to Anne of Cleves (1540) and Catherine Howard (1540–1542), maintaining proper court decorum while concealing her true feelings toward them with mixed results.[164] Under Henry's sixth wife, Catherine Parr (1543–1547),

Mary found some semblance of stability, sharing intellectual pursuits like translations of Erasmus. Catherine's Protestant leanings did clash with Mary's Catholicism, but their mutual respect endured. Mary's humanistic education shone through in her mastery of Latin and Greek, but her emotional scars caused her a lack of confidence. Where she was once a princess who glowed with happiness, her sad life had turned her into a reclusive and depressed young woman with chronic poor health.

Henry's death in 1547 transformed his only son into a king, with Mary named second in the succession under the Third Act of Succession (1544). Edward's Protestant regime, headed by Edward's maternal uncle the Duke of Somerset, left Mary marginalized and kept on the outside. Her traditional Catholic beliefs were seen as a threat to the stability of the new state religion, Protestantism. Mary defiantly flaunted Edward's religious reforms and held Mass at her estates in Essex and Norfolk, prompting rebukes from Edward's Privy Council, but Mary was determined to uphold her Catholicism at any cost. The stress of this familial and political rift caused her health to worsen, with fevers and pain noted by her household, causing her gynaecological problems to become even more debilitating. Mary's isolation grew, but her Spanish cousin, Emperor Charles V, offered her his support, urging her to stand firm in her religious beliefs.[165]

Edward's death on 6 July 1553, at 15, ignited a succession crisis. His Protestant advisors convinced the desperately ill young king to name his Protestant cousin Lady Jane Grey as the inheritor of his crown, bypassing Mary. When news of the succession reached Mary's ears, she rallied her supporters in East Anglia. Mary denounced Jane and declared herself queen at Framlingham Castle. 'She gathered a great force, and the people flocked to her'.[166] By July 19, Jane's regime quickly collapsed, and Mary entered London, her legitimacy affirmed by popular acclaim. Her health, however, remained precarious, with melancholy and weakness reported, hinting at the chronic ailments that had been plaguing her for decades.

Mary's first task as queen was consolidating power. She appointed loyalists like Stephen Gardiner, Bishop of Winchester, as Lord Chancellor, and relied on her Yorkist cousin, Cardinal Reginald Pole, for spiritual guidance. The Venetian ambassador praised Mary's 'prudent governance', as she balanced clemency with authority to secure her throne. But Mary's poor health, weakened by years of stress, was a permanent burden for her. Her courtiers cruelly gossiped about her weak constitution and bouts of depression. Mary's persistent ailments included headaches and irregular menstruation which depleted her strength and created doubts about if she could continue to reign without a strong king by her side.[167]

Mary's legitimacy rested on her father Henry VIII's will, but her Catholic faith alienated Protestant nobles. She moved carefully in her new role, releasing Catholic prisoners like the Duke of Norfolk and reinstating traditional Masses. She sought to avoid immediate confrontation with Protestants, knowing this would go against the will of her people. Her coronation on October 1, 1553, was a grand spectacle of continuity, held at Westminster Abbey with rituals codified by her grandmother, Margaret Beaufort. Predictably, her sex as a ruling queen was not looked upon with favour, as noted by Venetian ambassador Giovanni Michieli, who remarked that 'many doubt a woman's capacity to govern'.[168]

Mary hoped to restore Catholicism and reverse her brother's Protestant reforms. Her faith, which her mother instilled in her childhood, was unwavering. In 1553, she repealed Edward VI's Protestant laws, restoring the Mass and reinstating Catholic bishops like Stephen Gardiner. She sought papal reconciliation for England, dispatching envoys to Rome, although she faced resistance from nobility who had profited from the dissolved monasteries. Mary's religious policies alienated some members of her council, and sparked gossip with some in her court calling her a zealot. Her emotional reliance on her faith, drilled into her from childhood, drove her forward, but her melancholy deepened as civil resistance to her religious reforms grew.[169]

Mary's decision to marry her cousin Philip of Spain, the son of Emperor Charles V, was a critical moment for the new queen, aligning England with the Habsburg dynasty and its Catholic mission. As England's queen regnant, her Spanish choice of husband was fraught with political consequences. At the relatively advanced age of 37, Mary was forced to face the inevitable pressure to secure the succession and provide the realm with (male) heirs. Philip, eleven years her junior, was heir to Spain's vast empire, making the alliance another Habsburg triumph. Popular opinion was against the Spanish match, and several Privy Council members had their own doubts about the match as well.

Opposition culminated in Wyatt's Rebellion (January 1554), led by Sir Thomas Wyatt to depose Mary and prevent the Spanish match.

The rebels marched on London, but Mary's speech at the Guildhall rallied her subjects, 'She spoke with such courage that the city stood firm'. The rebellion collapsed, and Wyatt was executed. Mary's resolve hardened; emotional stake in the marriage, tied to her mother's Spanish heritage and her own desperate desire to secure a Catholic heir, drowned out the domestic opposition.[170]

On July 25, 1554, Mary wed Philip at Winchester Cathedral. Phillip was the first to arrive at the chapel, finely dressed in Mary's gifts of a white doublet and breeches with a mantle made entirely of cloth of gold. His robe was embroidered with jewels of every hue and pearls as well. The 37-year-old bride was wearing a gown of purple satin also embroidered with rich jewels and lined with purple taffeta. Her kirtle was white satin, embroidered in silver, and her train was carried by the Marchioness of Winchester. The cathedral was hung with cloth of gold for the occasion. The marriage initially bolstered Mary's reign, aligning England with the Habsburgs' anti-Protestant crusade and Philip's presence lent the realm credibility. His father, Charles V's support strengthened England's position against France. However, their personal dynamic was far from blissful. Mary thought she was deeply, passionately in love with her husband and positively showered him with affection; but Philip was detached, he preferred to focus on his Spanish and Imperial duties. He was courteous and distant with Mary and preferred spending his time on his correspondence with his father.[171]

In September 1554, mere weeks after her wedding to Philip on July 25, Mary summoned her physician to Whitehall Palace. Her voice was emotional with awe when she confided a secret: her monthly courses had ceased, a sign she feared trusting after years of menstrual difficulties. Dr Thomas Wendy, after examining her, confirmed her dearest wish – she was with child! He noted her cessation of monthly bleeding, morning nausea that left her pale, and a belly that was beginning to swell beneath her velvet gown. Spanish ambassador Simon Renard penned a fervent letter to Emperor Charles V, Philip's father: 'The Queen is with child, and all signs confirm it'.

'Bells rang through London, bonfires blazed, and the people rejoiced for the Queen's good news.' Mary I of England believed she was on the precipice of the fulfilment of her lifetime. Queen of England and wed to a Catholic prince, she now carried the kingdom's next Tudor heir in her womb. At 38, her body was worn down by decades of illness and her heart was scarred by childhood trauma. Despite her age and physical limitations she announced her pregnancy with joy. The whole realm rejoiced with their queen and the welcome rituals of impending motherhood commenced.[172]

Mary's face glowed with happiness, lifting the shadow of anxiety that had plagued her since childhood. Her ladies-in-waiting, Susan Clarencieux, Jane Dormer, Frances Waldegrave, and Mary Finch, admired her 'swollen womb', and helped Mary plan for her future child. Mary ordered Masses of thanksgiving in every cathedral, and couriers sped letters to Madrid, Vienna, and Lisbon, proclaiming the expected heir. At St Paul's Cathedral, Bishop Stephen Gardiner preached of a Catholic dynasty reborn, his voice ringing in triumph as crowds cheered 'God save the Queen's child!' Courtiers showered Mary with baby gifts: silver rattles, gold-stitched blankets, pearl-encrusted caps, and Mary and her women laboured over embroidered gowns for the royal layette. Mary, pious like her mother, knelt for hours in her chapel, her rosary held in her hands as she thanked the Virgin for this miracle. Philip put aside his usual emotional restraint and hosted lavish banquets in Whitehall's feasting hall, where both the Spanish and English nobles toasted the coming prince with wine and song. The kingdom eagerly awaited the birth of this new Tudor prince, no doubt seeing Mary's pregnancy as God's endorsement of her reign.

By November, Mary's condition continued to ripen. She moved between palaces; Whitehall to Greenwich, then Richmond, taking care to avoid strain, upholding Doctor Wendy's advice to rest in order to safeguard her pregnancy. Mary's nausea persisted past the usual first trimester, sometimes causing her to retire early, but she was reassured by her physicians that it was a common occurrence for a first-time mother. Her belly grew larger, pressing against her unlaced gowns, and she felt the 'quickening' or the baby's first movements which she described to Jane Dormer with a radiant smile.[173] Mary carefully followed the advice of her physicians, resting and making sure to eat whatever they prescribed. Nobility sent Mary ornate baby gifts and letters of congratulations, while the Privy Council drafted succession plans, naming the unborn child as Mary's heir. London's streets were atwitter with talk of a prince, and tavern keepers composed ballads to 'Mary's babe'. Habsburg Catholic allies rejoiced, and Charles V wrote to his son Philip praising this blessed union which would serve to strengthen Catholicism across Europe.

Mary's emotional investment in this pregnancy was profound. Her difficult childhood, marked by her parents' divorce, her mother's exile, and her own demotion, had left her determined to restore her mother's Catholic legacy. Her own regency demanded a successor, preferably male, to counter Protestantism. Mary felt both joy and anxiety as she tried to balance being queen with becoming a mother. She spent her evenings with Jane Dormer and Susan Clarencieux, planning her son's upbringing, envisioning a devout court steeped in Catholic virtue and Spanish culture. She commissioned a cradle adorned with Tudor roses and Habsburg eagles, blending the heir's dual heritage. The physicians calculated a spring birth, in May or June, and Mary planned an elaborate christening at Westminster Abbey, with Cardinal Reginald Pole to officiate. London's merchants decorated their shops with banners, and clergymen now preached of a new Catholic era, their sermons echoing Mary's faith.

In April 1555, Mary entered confinement at Hampton Court, adhering to the strict protocols set by her grandmother, Margaret Beaufort. Her chambers became a female-dominated sanctuary, decorated in crimson and gold tapestries that cloaked the walls and windows. A low fire warmed the confinement room's air against spring's chill. As dictated by protocol, only midwives and specially selected ladies could enter this space, creating a cocoon of protection for Mary, far from the worries of governance. Philip was barred by custom, so he lodged in nearby apartments, sending daily notes in his careful script, urging her to rest. A specially made silver cradle draped in velvet, and adorned with pearls waited to receive the newborn prince. Daily masses were said in honour of the queen in the palace chapel, with Mary's priests praying for a safe delivery.[174]

Mary rested on a cushioned bed, her belly now so big it strained against even her loosest gowns. She reported frequent movements to the delight of her midwives, who predicted a strong prince to honour Prince Philip. Doctor Wendy visited Mary twice daily, checking her pulse and prescribing gruel, light broths and herbal tonics. The court gathered outside of the confinement chambers and important personages like the Duke of Norfolk, Earl of Arundel, and Lord Paget arrived to witness the grand event. The Spanish Ambassador wrote to King Charles, telling him to expect a prince to unite England and Spain. Mary remained confined to her darkened rooms, she prayed and recited psalms, with her ladies gathered around her. She talked of naming the child Edward, after her brother, or Katherine, for her mother, her voice filled with hope. Her ladies embroidered baby clothes with Tudor roses, and the Privy Council prepared proclamations, envisioning a triumphant announcement. England held its breath, awaiting a Tudor-Habsburg heir, while the Habsburg courts in Brussels and Madrid sent envoys bearing gifts.[175]

Mary's due date came and went and still no labour. Doctor Wendy suggested Mary might have misjudged her dates. She remained hopeful, insisting that she felt the child move, her hands lovingly cradling her belly as she smiled at Doctor Wendy. Her ladies remained attentive, though some exchanged wary glances. June passed, and still no birth. Renard, the Spanish Ambassador's letters grew uneasy, noting 'her condition seems less certain'. Courtiers whispered of a false pregnancy, recalling Mary's lifelong ailments. The queen remained undeterred. She extended her confinement, her voice in prayer rising in anxiety and her rosary became a constant companion. Her Catholic faith sustained her, but the court's fervour waned, their enthusiasm fading away as summer loomed.

July came and still there was no child. Mary clung to hope, refusing to leave her confinement chambers, her prayers fervent, her rosary worn smooth by constant praying. Her ladies who usually gossiped merrily, now moved about the confinement rooms in muted horror, their eyes downcast. By late July, Ambassador Renard reported to Charles V that 'the Queen's belly diminishes', her condition 'doubtful'.[176]

Doctor Wendy confirmed no labour was imminent, and rumours of a mistake roiled through the court. In August, Mary emerged from Hampton Court with a sad and drawn face. Her belly was flat, her eyes heavy, and her spirit seemed broken. No royal proclamation explained the loss to Mary's puzzled subjects. Philip departed for the Netherlands a few days later, leaving Mary to face her sorrow alone. London's streets, once alive with song, grew quiet, the people's hope replaced by pity for their deserted queen. European courts sent cautious condolences, their envoys gossiping of England's misfortune.[177]

In January 1557, after Philip's brief return to England in 1556, Mary announced a second pregnancy. She called Doctor Wendy to Greenwich Palace, where he confirmed the familiar signs: no monthly courses, nausea that kept her in bed, and a swollen womb. Ambassador Renard, chastened by 1555, wrote cautiously to Charles V: 'Her Majesty believes herself with child', cautioning restraint until they could be certain. Mary's health was frailer than ever after years of emotional strain, yet her eyes shone with renewed hope. She ordered prayers across England, and churches rang their bells, though celebrations were decidedly muted, as subjects as well as courtiers recalled the earlier failure. Mary's conviction was unshaken – her heart was set on a Catholic heir to redeem her reign.[178]

Her court tried to muster up the expected enthusiasm, but experience had taught them to be wary. Mary's ladies-in-waiting complemented her on her swelling belly and once more they took up embroidery silks to begin on the new heir's layette. Mary limited her duties, resting at Greenwich in her chambers warmed by fires against the winter's chill. Her nausea became debilitating, forcing her to cancel audiences. Doctor Wendy told her that nausea was a good omen. She felt the quickening again and immediately shared her joy with Jane Dormer, who nodded with a strained smile. Ambassador Renard wrote of the great care she took to ensure a safe birth, presuming a spring delivery in April or May. The people offered cautious toasts, praying for a prince to ensure England's succession. Habsburg allies, though sceptical, sent messages of hope, eager for a Catholic heir to the Tudor throne.[179]

In March 1557, Mary entered confinement at Greenwich Palace, her chambers were transformed into a safe, cosy haven as before. Beautiful tapestries covered the walls, the windows were sealed, and the midwives prepared her bed with fresh linens. A select group of Mary's women attended her, distracting her with games of cards or busied themselves with folding swaddling cloths and baby clothes. Philip was abroad for much of the confinement period, but he sent letters from the Netherlands, reminding Mary to look after herself and be patient. All things were in readiness for the birth, including a cradle embellished with Tudor emblems waiting for its royal little inhabitant. Catholic Masses were held for Mary's safe delivery throughout the realm. Mary reported frequent movements within her womb, and her belly had been growing steadily.[180]

April arrived, but no labour followed. Mary insisted the child thrived; her faith buoyed her as she recited her rosary. Her ladies treated her with kindness, although privately they may have doubted the veracity of this pregnancy. Doctor Wendy reported no clear progress, and courtiers whispered of 'another false hope'. Mary's confinement stretched into May, her body weakening but her convictions remaining steadfast. Ambassador Renard wrote to Charles V of the queen's persistent abdominal swelling and her physical weakness. The court's attitude towards their sovereign was one of quiet dubiousness.[181]

May came in, but still there was no baby. Mary was heartbroken as she lingered in her dark confinement rooms, her prayers becoming desperate pleas, begging God to grant her a child. Her ladies were quiet and subdued as they served her reverently, though all knew no child was forthcoming. By June, the queen had left Greenwich in the same condition she entered it and she must have felt humiliated by her failed confinement. As before, there was no public acknowledgment of failure, nor explanation of what was happening with the queen's reproductive health. Mary's second hope had crumbled, leaving her to face another empty cradle amid mounting political strife, her heart heavy with unfulfilled duty. London's subjects again had their hopes for another Tudor heir crushed and European courts sent no further envoys.[182.]

Mary I's Unfulfilled Expectations

Mary I of England, crowned in 1553 and married to Philip of Spain in 1554, remained at the centre of a court waiting with anticipation for a Catholic heir. Her two announced pregnancies in 1554–1555 and 1557–1558 ignited fervent celebrations, prayers, and customary childbirth rituals, as she and her kingdom anticipated a Tudor-Habsburg child to secure her faith and dynasty. Sadly, no heir was born. The absence of a child raises the question: what happened during these pregnancies? Did Mary deliver stillborn infants, hidden by a court eager to protect her reputation? Did she give birth to live children who died soon after, their fates obscured by political necessity? Or were these pregnancies delusions, born of a body and mind strained by illness? I believe Mary deserves the benefit of a doubt, therefore, a thorough examination of the historical chronicles from Mary's time will be used to evaluate the possible outcomes of Mary's mysterious pregnancies.

One explanation for Mary's childless pregnancies is that she delivered stillborn infants, their deaths concealed to spare her public humiliation or to maintain political stability. In the sixteenth century stillbirths were not uncommon, especially for a woman of Mary's advanced maternal age of 38 in 1554 and 41 in 1557. A stillbirth is defined as the delivery of a foetus that dies in utero after twenty weeks. Could a stillborn baby or babies theoretically align with her reported symptoms? Amenorrhea, nausea, and a swollen belly were all noted by her physician, Dr Thomas Wendy, during both pregnancies. The court's elaborate preparations, including the set-up of nurseries, christening plans, etc., signify the genuine expectation of a baby, which could support the idea of a viable pregnancy. If Mary suffered a stillbirth, the midwives and physicians might have suppressed the news to avoid harming the queen's reputation or weakening her precarious reign, especially amid Protestant opposition and the Habsburg alliance's high stakes.

However, the historical record offers no evidence of stillbirths. During Mary's first pregnancy, announced in September 1554, she entered confinement at Hampton Court in April 1555, expecting a birth by May or June. The records detail the meticulous preparations: sealed chambers, an elaborate silver cradle, and daily Masses recited for a safe delivery. By July, Spanish ambassador Simon Renard observed a troubling change: 'The Queen's belly diminishes', and her condition was 'doubtful'. In August, she emerged from her confinement chambers, her abdomen flat, as Venetian envoy Giovanni Michieli saw with no mention of a baby having been delivered. Reportedly, the court felt a 'quiet shame' on behalf of their queen, but there is no mention whatsoever of a stillborn child. The absence of any reference to a birth – still or otherwise – is a significant omission in a court where every royal event, from baptisms to funerals, was meticulously documented. The much-mentioned Dr Wendy certainly would have made note of a royal birth, even if the outcome was not a desirable one. Midwives, such as those attending Mary, would have reported a stillbirth, and ladies-in-waiting, like Susan Clarencieux or Jane Dormer who were with Mary in her confinement, would have left some clue in their letters or in later accounts of a birth. The silence is deafening.

The second pregnancy, announced in January 1557, follows the exact same pattern. Mary entered confinement at Greenwich Palace in March, with preparations mirroring 1555: darkened chambers, an elaborate cradle, and the recitation of Masses for a safe birth. By May, Dr Wendy reported 'no clear progress', of the queen's pregnancy. In June, Mary emerged from confinement – without a baby. There is no public acknowledgment of a birth, only hushed disappointment. If a stillbirth had occurred, the court's secrecy would have been extraordinary, given the presence of dozens of attendants, physicians, and nobles expecting a public announcement. Spanish and Venetian ambassadors' letters contain no mention of a stillborn child, despite their detailed accounts of court gossip. Prince Philip, absent during much of 1557, received no report of a baby, born alive or not – this is significant proof that tragically, there never was a viable pregnancy.

Medical evidence further undermines the stillbirth theory. A stillbirth would of course involve labour, with physical signs like uterine contractions and the delivery of a foetus, yet no source mentions such events. Mary's reported 'quickening' (foetal movements) in both pregnancies could suggest a viable pregnancy, but her abdomen's regression in 1555 and lack of labour in both cases point away from a true pregnancy. Her chronic ailments, described as 'disorders of the womb' since her teens, suggest a gynaecological condition that could mimic pregnancy. The absence of any records of a burial, customary even for stillborn royal infants, as seen in Katherine of Aragon's losses, is more proof that no foetus existed. Furthermore, there is a void of material evidence – a coffin, a memorial, or a physician's report rules out a stillbirth.

Another possibility is that Mary gave birth to live children who died shortly after birth, but their deaths were concealed to protect her reign or the Habsburg alliance. In the sixteenth century, infant mortality was a common occurrence. A live birth could explain the court's elaborate preparations, from nurseries to christening plans, and the initial confidence of physicians like Wendy, who confirmed pregnancy signs in both 1554 and 1557. If a child was born alive but died soon after, Mary's attendants might have hidden the event to avoid public despair, political fallout, or Protestant propaganda claiming divine judgment as the cause for the babies' deaths. The omnipresent Habsburgs, in their eagerness for a Catholic heir, might have supported such secrecy to maintain England's alliance with Spain.

This scenario crumbles under scrutiny. The historical record lacks any evidence for a live birth. In 1554–1555, Mary's confinement at Hampton

Court stretched from April to August, with no delivery recorded by any midwife or physician or ambassador. The diminishment of the queen's belly by July was observed by all and sundry. Her emergence from confinement in August with a flat abdomen was recorded by foreign ambassadors. A live birth, even if the child had died immediately, would have required labour, attended by midwives and physicians, and certainly noted by Mary's women. The presence of dozens of attendants, yet none reporting a delivery or a child's death, cannot be ignored. Royal births, even tragic ones, were public events, with proclamations and ceremonies, as seen with Henry VIII's children by Katherine of Aragon.

The 1557–1558 pregnancy follows suit. Mary's confinement at Greenwich, from March to June 1557, ended without a birth. Once again, the queen emerges from her confinement with no mention of labour or a child. Ambassador Renard's letters, detailed on court matters, report only her 'sadness and weaknesses'. Dr Wendy's silence on a labour, birth, or death is also telling, as is the lack of any funeral or memorial, customary for all royal infants, even those babies who died soon after birth. The court's meticulous record-keeping, so meticulous in accounts of household expenses and diplomatic correspondence, would have recorded some trace of a child, living or dead. The absence of such records, despite the presence of foreign envoys and gossipy courtiers, makes a live birth implausible. Politically, concealing a live birth and death would have been risky. Mary's reign was already fragile amidst Protestant resistance and the loss of Calais. Mary needed public support for her Catholic restoration. A royal birth, even one followed by death, would have been a sixteenth-century sign of God's approval of her reign. Suppressing such an event would have served no purpose, especially when allies like Charles V and Cardinal Pole were urging her to strengthen her legitimacy. The Habsburgs were heavily invested in the alliance, and would have demanded a public announcement of a birth, however brief the child's life was. The silence from European courts, that eagerly awaited news of an heir, further undermines this theory. No source, English or foreign, hints at a living child, even in speculative gossip.

The third and most compelling explanation is pseudocyesis, a false pregnancy where psychological and physical factors mimic gestation. Mary's symptoms – amenorrhea, nausea, and a swollen belly, all align with pseudocyesis. In combination with her chronic gynaecological ailments, well known since her teens as 'The Mother' or 'suffocation of the matrix' paint a picture of reproductive dysfunction. These ailments, well documented by ambassadors like Eustace Chapuys in the 1530s, are consistent with endometriosis, a condition causing severe menstrual pain, irregular cycles, and ovarian cysts (endometriomas) that can cause abdominal swelling. Endometriosis could explain the physical signs mistaken for pregnancy, while pseudocyesis, driven by psychological factors (namely Mary's intense longing to present to Phillip a Catholic heir), explains the scenario of a false pregnancy.[183]

Mary desperately wanted a baby – for herself but more importantly, for the succession of her dynasty. Mary's history is overshadowed by tragedy. Her childhood was indelibly marked by her parents' divorce, her mother's exile, and her demotion, leaving Mary depressed and ill. Her desperate wish for an heir, inextricably tied to her Catholic mission and the pressures of the Habsburg alliance, caused intense psychological stress. The loss of Calais in 1558 and Philip's absences deepened her emotional distress. Pseudocyesis is caused by such turmoil, when desperate longing and stress trigger hormonal changes, like elevated prolactin and cortisol, producing symptoms like amenorrhea and abdominal swelling.[184] Mary's belief in her pregnancies was absolute, as seen in her joyous announcements and confinement rituals; sadly, the absence of labour or delivery in both cases points to a psychosomatic condition.

In 1554–1555, the regression of Mary's belly, observed by ambassador Renard as 'diminishing' by July, points to a distended uterus caused by endometriosis which eventually resolves; or a psychosomatic abdominal swelling which is common in pseudocyesis. By August, her abdomen was flat, as ambassador Michieli saw, with no signs of labour or a baby. The 1557–1558 pregnancy has an identical pattern, although the swelling persisted, as ambassador Renard noted, due to chronic endometrioma. No source mentions labour contractions, delivery, or a child, living or dead. The court's silence, the lack of burial records, and the absence of any physical evidence – such as a placenta or foetal remains – rules out actual gestation. Mary's physician was limited by his sixteenth-century knowledge, and misread her symptoms. Dr Wendy's reports of 'uncertain dates' and 'no clear progress' suggest a limited understanding of Mary's physical ailment. Her court, so eager for a Tudor heir, amplified Mary's delusion, they saw her symptoms through hope rather than scepticism. Endometriosis may cause symptoms like amenorrhea and abdominal swelling similar to pregnancy, while pseudocyesis can lead to nausea and perceived foetal movement due to hormonal and psychological factors. Mary's chronic endometriosis and emotional stress from desperately wanting children, marital pressure, and dynastic concerns led to her pseudocyesis.[185]

The absence of labour, burial, or any record whatsoever of a child in either pregnancy, despite the court's scrutiny, makes this the only scenario that fits the evidence.

The stillbirth and live birth scenarios, while plausible in theory, completely lack historical support. A stillbirth would have produced physical evidence – a foetus and a placenta, yet no source mentions such evidence. The court had extensively detailed records, including household accounts and diplomatic correspondence, so a birth would have been noted even if concealed. The absence of a burial or memorial was standard procedure for royal stillbirths, so this further refutes a stillbirth theory. A live birth followed immediately by the infant's death is even less likely, given the public nature of royal births. Had Mary given birth to a living child, an official declaration would have strengthened her authority, especially with Catholic Habsburg support for her successor. The lack of reports from courtiers, midwives, and envoys confirms the birth didn't take place.

Pseudocyesis, by contrast, explains the queen's symptoms, the court's belief, and ultimately, the absence of a child. Mary's endometriosis provided the physical signs – swelling, amenorrhea, and nausea that her mind, strained by trauma and dynastic pressure, interpreted as pregnancy. Her court was desperate for an heir, thereby reinforcing her delusion, as did physicians lacking modern diagnostics. The regression of symptoms in 1555 and their persistence in 1557–1558 align with pseudocyesis and endometriosis, not gestation, in my opinion. The historical record, with its stark silence on any birth, supports this conclusion.

Mary I's pregnancies of 1554–1555 and 1557–1558 were radiant visions that captivated her kingdom. From Whitehall's joyous tidings to Greenwich's silent despair, every detail – her swollen womb, her quickening, her darkened chambers – painted a portrait of motherhood. Yet no child was born. The theories of stillbirth or live birth, while possible in another context, find no evidence in the historical record, which lacks any trace of labour, delivery, or burial. Instead, pseudocyesis, caused by Mary's desperate maternal longings and compounded by endometriosis, explains the cruel absence of a royal birth. Her lifelong ailments and emotional wounds, rooted in a childhood of loss and intensified dynastic pressure, wove a mirage of motherhood. Mary's story, etched in the records of her time, reveals a queen whose body and soul, bound by illness and faith, conjured heirs that faded into shadows, leaving behind a legacy of sorrow.

Mary I of England, crowned in 1553 and wed to Philip of Spain in 1554, carried the weight of a kingdom's dreams and her own unyielding grief. Her reign was a fervent crusade to restore Catholicism, but it was marred by personal tragedy – childlessness, chronic illness, and an unfulfilling marriage caused by an absent and an unfeeling husband. By November 1558, at the age of 42, she lay dying in St James's Palace, her body weak and her spirit crushed by too many disappointed dreams. Her demise was due to 'dropsy' or 'melancholy'; unsatisfying and unscientific labels that fail to explain her death. I believe that Mary died of ovarian cancer, the culmination of a chain of events beginning with childhood trauma, which led to hormonal imbalances, leading to endometriosis, and ultimately, malignancy. Mary was a queen whose body and soul were ravaged by sorrow and sickness, until she succumbed to a silent, relentless disease.

Mary's early life was defined by loss, creating scars that shaped her health and reign. Born in 1516 to Henry VIII and Katherine of Aragon, she was a cherished princess, celebrated with feasts and pageants as England's heir. Her world began to crumble in the late 1520s when Henry sought to annul his marriage to Katherine in order to wed Anne Boleyn. By 1533, aged 17, Mary was declared illegitimate, stripped of her title, and banished to Hatfield House to serve her infant half-sister Elizabeth. Spanish ambassador Eustace Chapuys described her as grieving and melancholy, confined far from her mother, who died in 1536 at Kimbolton Castle, isolated and heartbroken. Courtiers noted Mary's distress – sleepless nights, loss of appetite, tearful outbursts, and fainting spells, all signs of profound emotional trauma. Her father's rejection, coupled with religious persecution as a Catholic in a shifting Protestant court, deepened her isolation. Chapuys' letters describe her distress at being kept from her mother, the Dowager Princess Katherine, and the growing pressure from her father and his advisers over her refusal to acknowledge Anne as the sole queen of England.

Specific events intensified Mary's suffering. In 1534, Henry's Act of Supremacy declared him head of the Church, forcing Mary to renounce her Catholic faith or risk treason. Her rejection of the situation resulted in house arrest and provoked her father's anger. In 1535, the execution of her mother's allies, like Bishop John Fisher, shook her resolve, as Chapuys noted her great fear for her own safety. These pressures, unrelenting and public, left her in a state of constant anxiety. Her physical health faltered, with reports of headaches, heart palpitations, and pain in her belly, as her governess, Margaret Pole, recorded in private letters. These pains, described as sharp and debilitating, forced her to stay in bed for days, disrupting her duties and alarming her household.

Modern medicine links childhood trauma to disruptions in the hypothalamic-pituitary-adrenal (HPA) axis, which regulates stress hormones like cortisol. Chronic stress like Mary endured, can elevate cortisol, suppress ovulation, and skew oestrogen levels, creating hormonal imbalances. Studies of early-life trauma show increased risks of gynaecological problems due to these disruptions. Mary's adolescence was marred by rejection and uncertainty, setting the stage for her later ailments. Her sixteenth-century physicians were unaware of these connections, noted her 'suffocation of the matrix' in 1535, a term used at the time for gynaecological ailments.[186]

Mary's lifetime of gynaecology complaints is very much aligned with the symptoms of endometriosis, a condition where tissue resembling the uterine lining grows outside the womb, causing severe pain, irregular periods, and often infertility.[187] It has been well documented that she suffered excruciating menstrual pain and erratic cycles, as documented by physicians and ambassadors alike. These symptoms, termed 'The Mother' or 'suffocation of the matrix', align with endometriosis, which does produce pelvic inflammation, adhesions, scarring, and ovarian cysts (endometriomas) that swell with blood, distending the abdomen. The queen's ladies – Jane Dormer, Susan Clarencieux, and Frances Waldegrave – were well aware of the severity of the queen's ailments. These pains sometimes left her bedridden for days, with sweating and faintness sometimes accompanying her agony.[188]

Sixteenth-century medical practices could offer her little relief, probably only exacerbating her suffering. Tudor era physicians were severely limited in their understanding of how the human body operates, their modus operandi was humoral theory. Humoral theory offered few treatment options other than bloodletting, or mercury-based tonics, which were ineffective or harmful. Dr William Butts suggested dietary changes – avoiding cold meats or spices – but these recommendations would have had little to no effect. Mary's condition remained untreated, chronicled by ambassadors who took notice of the toll it was having on the queen's health.[189]

Hormonal imbalances were to blame for the disorder, and these were not well understood in the sixteenth century. Mary's inability to conceive suggests infertility, a hallmark of endometriosis affecting up to fifty per cent of women suffering from this disorder. Her well-documented abdominal swelling also suggests endometriomas, which can distend the belly, causing visible bloating. Endometriosis is a condition that thrives in inflammatory environments, exacerbated by stress, which Mary endured to excess in her marriage and at court. These pressures intensified her symptoms, creating a vicious cycle of pain and emotional strain.

Women who suffer chronic endometriosis are two to three times more likely to get ovarian cancer as compared to the general population. Studies indicate that ongoing inflammation and hormonal imbalances may raise the probability of cancerous mutations, which can potentially transform benign endometriomas into malignant tumours. Mary's untreated condition, which existed from her teens to her forties, created such a risk, setting the stage for a deadly transformation.

By 1558, Mary's health had deteriorated alarmingly, painting a grim portrait of decline. Venetian and Spanish ambassadors described her as pale and thin with great weakness and persistent abdominal swelling that confined her to St James's Palace. They also remarked upon her sadness and 'debility', which led to the cessation of her public appearances. Her physicians, led by Dr Thomas Wendy and Dr John Calwood, reported swellings in her belly, feverish spells, weight loss, and profound fatigue. These symptoms are consistent with ovarian cancer, a disease often undetected until advanced. Unlike acute infections which kill swiftly, Mary's gradual decline over months suggests a malignancy. Ovarian cancer, particularly arising from endometriosis, fits her clinical picture. Untreated endometriomas may become malignant and pose serious risks.[190]

Mary's lifelong pelvic pain and abdominal swelling indicates she probably had cysts, which could have turned cancerous by her forties.[191]

The disease's diagnostic hallmarks – bloating, weight loss, and fatigue – match her symptoms very closely. Her feverish spells could be explained by tumour-related inflammation or infections, common in advanced stages. Her age (42) and childlessness (nulliparity) are risk factors, as epidemiology shows higher incidence in women who have never been pregnant.[192] Her physicians, lacking understanding of her disease, mistook her swelling for dropsy, a sixteenth-century term used for many conditions, but especially for severe bloating.

Mary's final months were marked by agony. By the summer of 1558, she was bedridden, suffering great pain and swollen limbs. Her daily life withered – she ceased attending Mass, a lifelong habit, and relied on Jane Dormer to read psalms to her. Her council, led by Cardinal Reginald Pole, prepared for Elizabeth's succession. Courtiers gossiped of a wasting sickness, spreading fear of an inexplicable decline. Mary began slipping into semi-consciousness by November, typical of cancer's terminal phase, with tumours spreading to the peritoneum, causing organ failure. Her death on November 17, 1558, followed weeks of decline – no sudden collapse but a steady fading away.

The theory that Mary I died as a result of ovarian cancer is supported by the preponderance of evidence beginning in her stressful childhood. The enormous amount of stress she experienced due to her parents' divorce and her mother's banishment disrupted her HPA axis, which caused elevated cortisol levels and the disruption of normal oestrogen production. This laid the groundwork for a life-long battle with endometriosis. Over the decades, blood-filled cysts formed and sparked a favourable environment for malignancies. Clearly there is a link between endometriosis and cancer. Historical records support this hypothesis. Eustace Chapuys' accounts of Mary's melancholic episodes as well as his notes on 'The Mother' all point to the symptoms which lead to Mary's fatal battle with ovarian cancer. The fact that Mary never had any pregnancies at all is another corresponding symptom of the theoretical diagnosis of ovarian cancer which is more prevalent in women who have never had children. This whole situation could have been avoided if only Henry had married her off at a reasonable age. Her heirs could have been placed in royal courts throughout Europe, continuing the Tudor line and creating a winning reproductive strategy. It's an unfortunate end to the reign of England's first queen regnant.

Chapter 6

The Last Queen's Orphan

I lay weak and ill; my tiny daughter mewling beside me in her lawn cap and gown, my tears sliding down the side of my face, onto her embroidered blanket. My poor darling, I am too weak to hold her. Thomas enters my chamber and is at my bedside, mumbling sweet words. Words of lies. Words of duplicity. I know that the very moment I am gone, he will go to her. He will ask her to be his wife and say those things mine own ears once heard. She won't be fool enough to believe him; she was always clever, that sly redheaded wench.

Catherine Parr, the woman who would one day marry a king, once led a quiet life of piety, intellectual curiosity, and modest ambition. Catherine was born into a gentry family; her mother gave her an uncommon education based on the early principles of humanism, not unlike Sir Thomas More's daughters had been given.

Catherine Parr was born around the year 1512, in her family's home in Blackfriars, a busy corner of London where the Thames undulated nearby and the air was thick with the chatter of merchants, courtiers, and scholars. Although historians like to romanticise her birth as happening at Kendal Castle in Westmorland, a nod to her family's northern roots, the evidence points to London. Blackfriars was the Parrs' base, a short distance from the heart of Tudor power where Catherine's mother served as a lady-in-waiting to Queen Katherine. She was the eldest child of Sir Thomas Parr and Maud Green, a couple who weren't fabulously wealthy but had the right connections to move in court circles. Thomas, a knight and courtier, had served Henry VII and Henry VIII. He collected lands and minor offices like stepping stones. Maud, meanwhile, served Queen Katherine of Aragon, Henry's first wife, the namesake of her eldest daughter.[193]

Catherine grew up with her younger siblings, William (born 1513) and Anne (born 1515); her two other siblings died in infancy, a tragic but common occurrence in Tudor England. The Parrs' Blackfriars house was no grand palace, but it was a lively place with servants hauling firewood, visitors telling tales of court intrigues, and an occasional scholar arriving with wonderful new books bound in leather. Catherine, with her love of books and her quick mind, was right in the middle of the action, absorbing the rhythms of a household tied to the court.

When Catherine was about 5, life dealt her a devastating blow. Her father died in 1517, possibly from the sweating sickness, a dreadful disease that could snatch a man's life away in just hours. Lady Maud was only 25 years old, and her husband's death left her a widow with three young children and a family name to uphold. She could have remarried to secure her future as most widows did, but Maud chose a different path. She managed the lands and tenants and continued to acquire court connections with resolve. For young Catherine, watching her mother run the show was like witnessing a master at work. Maud wasn't just keeping the family afloat; she was building a legacy, demonstrating to her daughter what it meant to be a strong woman in a century that rarely gave women the ability to do so. Those early years in Blackfriars were filled with music, learning, and feminine ambition which would plant the seeds of resilience and curiosity in Catherine's life.[194]

Maud Green wasn't content to raise her children as mere ornaments for court. The Renaissance was sweeping through Europe, bringing with it humanist ideas about learning, reason, and virtue, and Maud wanted her children to benefit from it. While most girls of the gentry learned just enough to recite prayers and embroider a neat sampler, Catherine got an education that was practically revolutionary. Maud ensured that her daughter could read and write in English and Latin, as well as French. This humanist education was not about showing off; it was about developing a mind that could think critically and hold its own in a world dominated by men.

Maud's Renaissance-style vision for Catherine went far beyond books. She taught her the skills that would set her above other girls in her socio-economic class: dancing with grace to charm her beaux, playing the lute to elicit sighs from a room, and stitching beautiful embroidery that told stories in thread. And of course, managing a household down to the last barrel of ale. These were the survival tools in a society where marriage was a woman's means of security and influence. Maud and her daughter would pore over household accounts together, with Maud showing Catherine how to negotiate with a stubborn merchant or soothe an irritable tenant. It was a hands-on education in leadership, disguised as domesticity. Religion was woven into Catherine's learning, too, and the Renaissance was a wild time for faith. Martin Luther's ideas were shaking the Catholic Church to its core, sparking debates that echoed even in England's quietest corners. Catherine grew up in a traditional Catholic household, steeped in the rituals of Mass and confession, but her humanist studies honed her mind for deeper questions. What did faith really mean? Was it about following the priest's every word or finding a personal connection to God? As a teenager with a sharp mind, those early questions were like sparks, waiting for the right moment to ignite into the religious passion that would define her later years.[195]

By her late teens, Catherine's life took the turn every Tudor girl expected: marriage. In 1529, when she was about 17, Maud arranged for her to wed Sir Edward Borough, son of Thomas, 3rd Baron Borough of Gainsborough, a Lincolnshire family with land and a title. It wasn't a love match but a strategic one, tying the Parrs to a respected northern family. Edward wasn't the heir – his older brother had that title – but this marriage was a solid step up for the Parrs. Catherine packed her belongings and moved to Kirton-in-Lindsey, a modest manor in Lincolnshire's green countryside. For a girl raised in London's lively Blackfriars, it must have felt like stepping into a quieter, slower world, where the days were marked by the rhythm of harvests and the births of newborn livestock.[196]

Catherine's husband Edward was young, perhaps in his early twenties, but frail, possibly battling a chronic illness that sapped his strength. Their marriage wasn't a romantic love-match, it was a practical alliance, meant to boost the Parrs' social standing. Catherine immersed herself into her role as lady of the house, quickly learning the nuts and bolts of estate management – overseeing servants, balancing budgets and ensuring that the larder was stocked. It wasn't glamorous work, but she was good at it, her practical nature shining through even at 17.

The marriage was short-lived. Edward died around 1533, leaving Catherine a widow at approximately 21 years old. They had no children, and she was left with little more than a few years of experience and a new kind of independence. Widowhood was a strange place – part freedom, part uncertainty. Without a husband, Catherine had a taste of autonomy, but she was also vulnerable and reliant on her family for support without a husband to protect her. She returned to Blackfriars, leaning on her mother's wisdom to navigate this new phase. Those brief years as Lady Borough were a crash course in practicality, teaching Catherine how to keep a household running and hold her head high when life didn't go as planned.[197]

Catherine didn't stay as a widow for long. In 1534, at about the age of 22, she married John Neville, 3rd Baron Latimer, a widower nearly twice her age with a title, wealth, and a sprawling castle called Snape in Yorkshire. This was a big leap up the social ladder, arranged by her uncle William Parr, who had connections in the north. Catherine traded Lincolnshire's gentle fields for Yorkshire's wild, windswept moors. Snape Castle was a stone fortress that was both grand and isolated. It was a far cry from London's buzz, but Catherine stepped into her new role with confidence and an ability for making things work.

John Neville had two children from his first marriage, John, aged 14, and Margaret, aged 9; and Catherine became their stepmother. She wasn't the cold, distant figure of fairy tales, by all accounts she was a warm and engaging stepmother, building a genuine bond with the children. Margaret, in particular, seems to have looked up to her, and Catherine's care for her stepchildren shaped a nurturing side of her that would come into play later in her marriage to the king. Running Snape Castle was no small feat; she had to organise feasts for visiting nobles and ensure that the harvest was stored. She kept the castle's defences ready too, in a region known for its unrest. Catherine's days were full, from checking the kitchens to reviewing accounts with the steward, her skills earning her respect in a household that could have been tough to win over.

Yorkshire wasn't a peaceful retreat. The 1530s were a turbulent time, with Henry VIII's break from the Catholic Church splitting England in two. John Neville was a devout Catholic, and Yorkshire was a stronghold of those who clung to the old faith, wary of the king's new Church of England. In 1536, the Pilgrimage of Grace erupted – a massive rebellion of northerners demanding a return to Catholicism. Catherine's husband John was caught in a dangerous spot; he was loyal to the king but suspected of sympathising with the rebels. At one point, Snape Castle was overrun by armed rebels, and Catherine, barely in her mid-twenties, found herself in the middle of a very dangerous situation. She didn't crumble – she couldn't afford to. That experience was like fire hardening iron, teaching her how to stay composed when the world turned chaotic.[198]

The rebellion was crushed, but it left scars. The north remained restless, and John's health began to falter in the early 1540s. By March 1543, he had passed away, leaving Catherine a widow again at the age of around 31. This time, she walked away with a substantial inheritance – lands, money, and a wealth of experience. Her years as Lady Latimer had made her a past mistress at running a noble household, navigating religious tensions, and keeping cool in a crisis. She'd seen the raw edge of Tudor politics, from whispered plots to outright rebellion, and she'd come out stronger for it.

After John's death, Catherine didn't linger in Yorkshire. She returned to London, probably staying with her mother or her sister Anne, who was married to William Herbert, a rising Tudor courtier. London was teeming with glittering banquets, whispered schemes, and … ambition. Catherine was now a wealthy widow in her early thirties, and a good catch. She was educated, poised, and battle-tested, with a quiet strength that made people take notice. In late 1542 or early 1543, Catherine Parr, a widowed noblewoman, entered the household of Princess Mary as a lady-in-waiting, a role that thrust her into the heart of the Tudor court. Catherine's entry into Mary's household was facilitated by her family's entrenched connections. Catherine's siblings were active at court: her brother, William Parr was created Earl of Essex, and her sister, Anne Parr, had served as a lady-in-waiting to Henry's queens, including Jane Seymour and Catherine Howard. Anne's marriage to William Herbert, a courtier with ties to the royal family through his sister's marriage into the Howard clan, further strengthened the Parrs' influence. These connections lead to Catherine's introduction to Mary's circle, through William's advocacy or Anne's connections within the queen's household, which overlapped with Mary's during court gatherings.[199]

The timing of Catherine's widowhood in March 1543 was critical. Freed from her duties as Lady Latimer, she was available to relocate to London or to a nearby royal residence, making her a prime candidate for court service. While Mary's Catholic faith made her a focal point for conservative factions, her household required ladies who could balance piety with discretion in a court increasingly influenced by Protestant ideas. Catherine's northern background, rooted in Yorkshire's Catholic strongholds, aligned with Mary's conservative beliefs, while her reputation for tact made her a solid choice, despite her private leanings toward reformist theology.

As a lady-in-waiting, Catherine's duties included attending Mary during court functions, such as banquets or religious services, managing her wardrobe of elaborate gowns, organising entertainments like musical performances, and participating in her daily devotions, which centred on Catholic masses. She travelled with Mary between residences, ensuring her household ran smoothly, and engaged in the delicate task of representing Mary's interests in a court where religious tensions existed beneath the surface. Catherine's poise, intellect, and maturity, qualities honed through years of managing a noble household, distinguished her among younger and less experienced ladies. By early 1543, her presence in Mary's circle had caught the attention of Henry VIII, who was seeking a new queen after the execution of Catherine Howard in February 1542, setting the stage for a life-altering proposal.[200]

In the spring of 1543, Henry VIII, aged 51, was a diminished figure. He was obese with stinking leg ulcers and an unstable temperament. The execution of Catherine Howard for adultery had left him humiliated; now he sought a queen to restore stability, provide companionship and soothe his ruffled ego. His wandering eye fell upon Catherine, who had set her sights on a far more virile and handsome young man. Thomas Seymour, a charming, ambitious courtier with ties to the royal family through his late sister, Queen Jane Seymour, was more than happy to engage with Catherine. Their infatuation began heating up, a spark of something personal in a life previously shaped by duty. But unfortunately for Catherine, Henry had made up his mind. Her intellect, experience, and court connections were exactly what he needed. Her life before 1543 wasn't a fairy tale, it was real, raw, and full of hard lessons. She'd lost a father, buried two husbands, faced down rebels, and cultivated a mind that could hold its own in any room. She was a woman who'd learned to survive, to think, and to lead. She was ready to become queen whether she wanted to be or not. Her true love, Thomas Seymour, would not become her next husband, for when the king stretched out his hand to you, you had no choice but to take it.[201]

On July 12, 1543, Catherine Parr stood in the intimate Queen's Closet at Hampton Court Palace, its walls draped with luxurious tapestries, as she married King Henry VIII. The ceremony was understated, with fewer than twenty guests including Princess Mary, Princess Elizabeth, and courtiers like Archbishop Thomas Cranmer. They bore witness to a union heavy with expectation. Catherine's chosen motto, 'To be useful in all I do', was more than a phrase; it was a pledge to make the best of a treacherous role as queen with the wisdom and poise she had cultivated over years of life amongst members of the peerage. From that summer day until Henry's death on January 28, 1547, Catherine's queenship was a balancing act, managing her roles of consort, stepmother, nurse, regent, and religious reformer. In a court full of intrigue and led by a king frail in body and unstable in his temperament, she brought stability, intellect, and compassion, leaving a lasting mark on the Tudor dynasty's final years under Henry VIII.

Catherine's tenure as queen, from July 1543 to January 1547, tested her resilience and ingenuity. Unlike Henry's earlier wives, chosen for fertility, beauty, or dynastic alliances, Catherine was a companion for his declining years, tasked with easing the burdens of a king whose health was failing. At 51 when they married, Henry was no longer the swaggering young monarch who had once dazzled Europe. He was a very sick man with chronic leg ulcers emitting a stench so pungent that ambassador Eustace Chapuys called it 'noisome'. It caused him relentless pain, resisting even the most skilled physicians. By 1546, his weight – perhaps exceeding 300 pounds – confined him to specially crafted chairs or wheeled litters, in order to make movement through palaces like Whitehall or Hampton Court possible. And then there was his temperament which was erratic and often frightening, causing his courtiers to be constantly on guard.[202]

Catherine rose to the challenge of nursing Henry with a blend of practical care and emotional insight – in modern parlance she would be someone who possessed 'emotional intelligence'. She worked closely with Henry's physicians who applied poultices of herbs and linen to reduce the ulcer's swelling and prescribed tonics to dull the king's pain. Catherine adopted careful oversight of Henry's diet, choosing wholesome foods to avoid worsening his frail health. She spent long hours in his private apartments, where the air was thick with the stench of his leg wounds. Catherine also understood that Henry's needs extended beyond the physical; she engaged him in conversations about poetry, a pastime he still cherished, reading him verses to lift his spirits. Music, a passion they both shared, became a vital distraction. She arranged for a variety of musicians to perform for the king in his private chambers, briefly transporting him from his suffering.[203]

Her daily life as queen was a demanding list of responsibilities, challenging her skills at managing both people and their expectations. Her mornings often began in Henry's chambers, where she oversaw his medical care, consulted with physicians, and shared a modest breakfast with him while discussing court business. She then retreated to her own apartments where she managed a household of over 100 servants – maids, cooks, grooms, and chaplains. Her wardrobe was a significant undertaking, but one she loved. Her selections of gowns in velvet, cloth-of-gold, or damask were carefully chosen to protect an image of queenship, worn to assert authority at court gatherings. She seemed to love fashion and made unusual choices which are reflected in portraits of her at the time.

Evenings allowed Catherine to showcase her talent as the court's hostess, arranging entertainments that upheld Henry's image as a powerful monarch despite his physical decline. She held elaborate banquets and masques which were performances enacting tales of chivalry, loyalty, or classical virtues, accompanied by painted backdrops and flickering torchlight. Catherine occasionally joined in the dancing, showcasing her graceful beauty, though Henry could only sit and observe as his health made dancing impossible now. These events, attended by ambassadors from Spain, France, or the Holy Roman Empire, served as diplomatic propaganda, reinforcing England's prestige. Ambassadors acknowledged and praised Catherine's ability to maintain the court's grand facade, a testament to her skill in managing a dangerous political stage with a sickly, unstable monarch at its helm.[204]

Catherine's role as stepmother was one she treasured; she showed genuine care for Henry's three children: Mary, aged 27, Elizabeth, 9, and Edward, 5. Each child suffered because of their mothers' unfortunate fates – Katherine of Aragon's annulment, Anne Boleyn's execution, and Jane Seymour's death after childbirth, compounded by Henry's unpredictable favour. Catherine's motherly compassion and diplomatic tact helped to mend these fractures. For Edward, the Tudor heir, she took charge of his education. She engaged tutors like John Cheke who taught

Edward Protestant theology, Latin, and Greek to prepare him for the throne. She visited his household at Hertford, bringing him little gifts like illuminated manuscripts or carved wooden toys, and her loving care gave Edward a much-needed sense of warmth and stability.[205]

With Elizabeth, Catherine recognised a girl who desperately needed a mother and Catherine began a close relationship with her. At 9 years old, Elizabeth was brilliant with a passion for languages and religion, just like Catherne herself. Catherine encouraged her to learn with gifts of books as well as many precious hours spent conversing with her about religion. This early introduction to debate kindled Elizabeth's lifelong love of intellectual pursuits. Mary, at 27, proved to be a much more difficult challenge for Catherine due to her rigid Catholicism, which clashed with the queen's reformist tendencies. Yet Catherine managed to maintain a respectful relationship with Mary, attending Catholic masses with her, while quietly pursuing her own Protestant learning. Her diplomacy was pivotal in the 1543 Succession Act, which restored Mary and Elizabeth to the line of succession.[206]

Catherine transformed her household into a hub of intellectual and religious discussions, reflecting her love for learning. In 1545, she published *Prayers or Meditations,* the first book by an English queen under her own name. This collection of devotions, emphasising personal faith over Catholic rites, was carefully worded not to offend Henry's conservative doctrines, disguising her reformist leanings. She started writing *The Lamentation of a Sinner* during this marriage, a work that revealed her Protestant convictions, though she wisely delayed its publication until after Henry's death. Her private apartments became a gathering place for scholars and lovers of the Reformation. By candlelight, they discussed the great theological questions – whether salvation came through faith alone and should scripture be accessible in English to the public. These conversations carried risk in a court sensitive to religious dissent. Catherine supported Cranmer's liturgical reforms and advocated for the distribution of English prayer books among her household, furthering the cause of reform at court.[207]

In 1544, Catherine's responsibilities expanded exponentially when Henry embarked on a military campaign in France to capture Boulogne, leaving her as queen regent from July to September. Her management was remarkably competent and poised. Working with a council led by Thomas Cranmer, she oversaw the realm's finances, ensuring funds for the war effort. She also coordinated combat supplies for the kingdom's warriors, barrels of salted meat, and bundles of arrows. She also adeptly handled England's defences against potential Scottish raids along the northern border. To maintain court morale, she hosted grand entertainments, such as feasts for the Imperial ambassadors, featuring music, singing, and poetry recitations. Her deportment reinforced England's stability in Henry's absence.[208]

Catherine's reformist activities came to light in the summer of 1546, and they nearly proved her undoing. Henry's break with Rome in 1534 had created a divisive religious atmosphere, with traditional Catholics like Bishop Stephen Gardiner and Chancellor Thomas Wriothesley pitted against reformists like Thomas Cranmer. As Supreme Head of the Church of England, Henry enforced a conservative doctrine and was wary of Protestant radicalism. Catherine's theological discussions, particularly her association with Anne Askew, who was arrested and executed for heresy in July 1546, provided fodder for her enemies. Gardiner and Wriothesley accused her of heresy, citing her gatherings and writings as evidence of dangerous beliefs. A warrant for her arrest was prepared, and her books, including *Prayers or Meditations*, were used as evidence against her for her Protestant leanings.[209]

Forewarned, possibly by Dr Wendy, Henry's personal physician, or a sympathetic courtier, or a loyal member of her household, Catherine acted innocent. She approached Henry in his private apartments, kneeling in a gesture of humility; she described her contentious discussions as efforts to divert his mind from pain. She insisted that she gained from his 'learned discourse', insisting that she had no intention of challenging his authority. Her words, delivered with exaggerated submission, appealed to Henry's ego. Moved, he declared them good friends once more. When Wriothesley arrived the next day to arrest her, Henry rebuked him sharply, calling him a beast and a knave. The plot against the queen collapsed, and Catherine emerged unscathed, her quick thinking and diplomatic finesse critical assets of survival in a treacherous court.[210]

By 1546, Henry's health had deteriorated significantly. His leg ulcers got worse and caused him relentless pain, and his obesity made mobility nearly impossible. Catherine's nursing became increasingly critical, involving coordination with physicians, oversight of his restricted diet, and efforts to lift his spirits through conversation and music. By January 1547, his condition was dire. On January 28, 1547,

Henry died at Whitehall Palace, aged 55. His final hours were closely guarded, with only a few trusted courtiers, at his bedside. His death was briefly concealed to ensure a smooth transition to Edward's reign. Henry's will, finalised in December 1546, named Edward as heir, with Mary and Elizabeth restored to the succession, a reflection of Catherine's influence in unifying the royal family. As dowager queen, she retained significant wealth, including estates like Chelsea Place and Hanworth. Thomas Seymour was ready and willing to take up where they had left off before Catherine's marriage to Henry. Thomas had proposed marriage to 13-year-old Princess Elizabeth in February 1547 and had been rejected, so Catherine was the next best match for a social climbing, power hungry Seymour. The whole court had been gossiping about Thomas Seymour's ambitious plans to marry up – there is even speculation he may have proposed to Princess Mary as well. When his plans to marry into the succession were met with rejection, he settled on the next most important woman in England, Catherine Parr. Throwing caution to the wind, Catherine married Seymour without King Edward's approval in a secret ceremony in May 1547. Fewer than a dozen attended – Catherine's sister Anne Parr, a few loyal ladies, and a trusted chaplain, all swearing secrecy to avoid the Privy Council's scrutiny. Marrying so soon after Henry's death, barely four months, was a bold act; Tudor custom demanded widows, especially royal ones, wait at least a year to avoid scandal. Catherine, guided by love and perhaps a desire to reclaim her life, risked disapproval, believing Seymour shared her vision of a home built on affection and faith.

The marriage, though, sparked immediate controversy, most notably from young King Edward VI. At 9, Edward was a serious, smarmy little boy steeped in Protestant theology and already showing signs of his father's narcissism. However, he was genuinely fond of Catherine, who had nurtured him as a stepmother, visiting his household at Hertford with gifts of books or toys and ensuring his education prepared him for kingship. Thomas approached King Edward, and being only 9 years old, Edward was easily manipulated by his uncle into thinking he himself had come up with the idea of Thomas marrying Catherine. The king's Privy Council was not amused by Uncle Thomas' brash actions and tensions arose between the Lord Protector and the newlyweds.[211]

King Edward, once he fully understood what had taken place between Catherine and Thomas in direct violation of court protocol, became distant and cold toward both his uncle and his stepmother. The council, led by the Lord Protector, imposed a fine on Thomas Seymour for marrying without permission, a public rebuke that stung Catherine's pride. There was one other person deeply offended by this marriage – Princess Mary who never forgave Catherine for this perceived slight to her late father's memory.[212]

Catherine made her household at Chelsea, and brought Princess Elizabeth there to live with her and Seymour. She finally had a place where she could practice her Protestantism unchecked and in November 1547, she published *The Lamentation of a Sinner*, a work that urged a personal connection to God. Her rooms, warmed by fires and hung with embroidered tapestries, hosted debates on scripture and salvation, much like the humanist circles her mother, Maud Green, had introduced her to decades earlier. Princess Elizabeth, aged 13, thrived in this environment, her thirsty intellect devouring Latin, Greek, and theology under tutors hand-picked by Catherine herself.[213]

But beneath this scholarly decorum, something else was brewing. Thomas Seymour, now lord of the household, had free reign to do as he pleased. His ambition burned bright; he chafed at his brother's dominance as Lord Protector and saw Catherine's wealth and Elizabeth's royal status as tools to climb up higher on the social ladder. Feeling secure in his own sheltered world he now had the time and opportunity to indulge his whims.

Elizabeth, at 13, was a striking figure – tall, fair-skinned, with red-gold hair and a wit that proved her royal blood. Under Catherine's care she flourished, translating French texts and debating scripture with a fervour that echoed Catherine's own. But Seymour's presence disrupted this harmony. Beginning in the spring of 1547, he took to stealing into Elizabeth's chambers early in the morning, often clad only in his nightshirt. He then crawled into bed with Elizabeth and slapped her on the buttocks and teased her with inappropriate remarks, framing it as jest. Elizabeth, caught completely off guard, would try to escape, her discomfort masked by nervous giggles. To modern eyes, these actions are unequivocally inappropriate, a predatory abuse of power by a man in his late thirties toward a 13-year-old girl under his guardianship. Even in the Tudor era, where physical familiarity was common in noble households, Seymour's behaviour breached the decorum expected of a stepfather and a man of his rank, especially toward a princess second in line to the throne. Kat Ashley, Elizabeth's governess, brought these early morning visits to the attention of Catherine.

Catherine's initial response was shaped by her love for Seymour. She seemed to see his actions as playful, perhaps a clumsy attempt to bond with his stepdaughter. Bizarrely, she began accompanying Thomas on these escapades, abetting his inappropriate attentions toward Elizabeth. One incident, recorded in the 1549 depositions, occurred in Chelsea's garden, where Catherine held Elizabeth while Seymour, laughing, took out his dagger and shredded her dress into 100 pieces. The act left Elizabeth humiliated and confused. At 13, she was old enough to sense the impropriety but too young to fully challenge it. Kat Ashley noticed how Elizabeth began arising very early in the morning so that when Seymour entered her bedchamber she was already dressed. However, Elizabeth also seemed drawn to Thomas' charisma, a dangerous pull for a girl in her position. Ashley, alarmed, tried to intervene, urging Seymour to stop, but he dismissed her, insisting it was mere play. These encounters escalated and rumours of the inappropriate relationship between Thomas Seymour and Elizabeth reached the ears of people outside of Chelsea.[214]

By early 1548, Seymour's morning visits and intimate jests had become too frequent, too bold. A pivotal moment came when Catherine reportedly found them in an embrace and it finally triggered something inside Catherine, shattering her illusions of a harmonious marriage. The incident, noted in later depositions, marked a turning point. Catherine, who had navigated Henry's court with finesse, recognised the danger to Elizabeth's reputation and her own standing as dowager queen. In May 1548, she made the heart-wrenching decision to send Elizabeth away to live with her friends Sir Anthony Denny and his wife Joan at Cheshunt, a move that protected the princess but strained their bond. Catherine's care for Elizabeth, so tender during Henry's reign, was tested by this necessity, a painful reminder of the cost of her marriage to Seymour.

Seymour's behaviour toward Elizabeth was part of a broader pattern of reckless ambition combined with poor judgment that strained his marriage to Catherine. He saw Elizabeth as a means of getting closer to the crown, her status as a potential heir a glittering prize. His flirtations, however inappropriate, were laced with calculation, perhaps he even fantasised about how to use her to win the throne. He would have to postpone his delusions of grandeur because Catherine was pregnant and at the age of 35 or 36, it was likely to be a difficult time for her.

Sudeley Castle in Gloucestershire was selected by Catherine and Thomas to be the place for their child to be born. Situated in a picturesque valley at the foot of the Cotswold Hills and surrounded by gardens and parkland, it was a serene place to have a baby. Catherine decorated the nursery in her favourite colours of red and gold and waited patiently for the day of the baby's birth to arrive.[215]

On August 29, 1548, Catherine went into labour. Very little details are available on what happened during labour but as a midwife I can try and fill in some of the missing pieces. Catherine sadly died of puerperal fever five days after giving birth, and this detail is critical in trying to piece together what may have transpired during labour. A primipara or a first-time mother at the age of 36 in Tudor times would be more likely to have difficulty during labour than, say a 20-year-old would have. She may have even been 37, because her exact date of birth is not known. A straightforward birth would result in causing the death of the mother, but somehow bacteria was introduced into the birth canal probably after the sac of water broke, leading to infection. I imagine that Catherine may have been labouring with a baby who had a mal presentation – possibly *occipital posterior* where the baby's face is 'sunny side up'. This could explain why there was intervention in the labour process as this causes uneven dilation of the cervix. The baby's head in this position puts uneven pressure on the mouth of the womb, and if this is what happened, it was common practice at this time to manually dilate the cervix; the midwife would insert her fingers and pull open the womb to get the baby out. This would undoubtedly cause infection. There are other possibilities, but this one seems the most plausible explanation given the age of the mother and the subsequent death caused by a uterine infection. Catherine was alive only a few days to enjoy her daughter and at the end of her life she bitterly excoriated her husband Thomas for his ill treatment of her. It was a tragic ending for such a great queen.[216]

Chapter 7

The Other Woman: Royal Mistresses and Their Illegitimate Offspring

The goal of a royal dynasty is to forge alliances, conquer territory and reproduce as many heirs as possible. Queens can only do so much; even a very fertile queen can only have a limited number of children, but a king can father dozens if he isn't limited to one woman exclusively. Having a mistress was not only socially acceptable for a king, but it was also expected, and mistresses could aid the queen too, by diverting gossiping and criticisms away from her like a lightning rod. In times of infertility or recurrent still births, a king' mistress might reassure the court of the king's virility. Yet this also heightened the pressure on the queen to deliver an heir; the mistress it could be said exists in a paradox. She is a rival and also a protector undermining and supporting the queen simultaneously.

The French in particular had a custom of raising a mistress to an elevated status. The *maîtresse-en-titre* title offered a woman many of the same benefits a queen had: royal apartments, beautiful jewels and clothes, and her children had a nearly royal status, often raised to become members of the peerage. While French mistresses had this unique status, it was less socially accepted in English courts, but certainly just as common. There are many examples of mistresses in the Plantagenet, Lancastrian and Tudor royal houses. Women like Katherine Swynford, whose passionate affair with John of Gaunt birthed a dynasty, or Elizabeth Blount, whose son nearly altered Tudor succession. These affairs were not mere scandals; they changed the trajectory of England's future. Across the northern border, the mistresses of Scotland's James IV, like Janet Kennedy and Margaret Drummond, gave birth to children who grew up to have a hand in shaping Scottish history. The mistresses of the kings of England are in some cases largely forgotten, but they served an important role in the broader context of successful reproductive strategies.

Within history's shadowy perimeters lived the midwives who served both the queens and the mistresses. These women had to be highly skilled and also very discreet; a baby caught in the wee hours of the morning might grow up to be a nobody or that child might one day upend the dynasty. A trusted midwife was a crucial but silent player in the Wars of the Roses and in many a scandal that followed. She alone might know whether a child was a royal heir or an illegitimate bastard. It was the midwife who hid a dead baby or secretly spirited it away. These women kept the kingdom's most closely guarded secrets. They watched the rise of bastards they delivered, like Henry FitzRoy, or perhaps they organised quiet disappearances of children whose paternity had the potential to threaten the crown. They administered abortifacients, delivered dead or disfigured babies in silence, and if necessary, buried the evidence with their own hands. Their loyalty was never publicly rewarded, but their betrayal could have the power to rewrite history. In every whispered rumour about a hidden child, there was a midwife who knew the truth, and yet their names are almost never recorded. Their lives existed just outside of the official chronicles, but without them, the royal family tree might look very different.

In some rare cases, the mistress did not remain in the shadows, although usually her midwife did. Sometimes this mistress in the dynastic narrative became central, even celebrated. No woman illustrates this better than Katherine Swynford, whose long and scandalous love affair with John of Gaunt, Duke of Lancaster would eventually become a legal marriage. The children born of their affair named Beaufort after the area where John of Gaunt owned vast lands were not royal bastards exiled into obscurity. They were woven directly into the fabric of the English Crown. Katherine's story offers one of the most striking examples of a mistress whose womb reshaped royal history; from her lineage would come Margaret Beaufort, and through her, Henry VII, founder of the Tudor Dynasty, What began as a private passion became a public bloodline, and if the rumours are true, her births were attended quietly and discreetly in the care of a trusted woman whose name has not survived, but whose work would echo through the centuries.

Katherine Swynford: The Mistress Turned Queen

One of the mistresses who had perhaps the biggest impact on England's royal dynasty was Katherine Swynford. She was born around 1350 in Hainaut, a lush land of winding rivers and busy markets in what is now known as Belgium. Her father, Paon de Roet, was a knight in the service of Queen Philippa, Edward III's consort. He is responsible for giving his family a foothold in the dazzling orbit of England's royal court. By 1390, at the age of 40, Katherine had become the mistress of John of Gaunt, Duke of Lancaster, one of England's most powerful figures at this time. Katherine's love affair with Gaunt, a man whose impressive wealth and influence rivalled that of many kings, produced four children – John, Henry, Thomas, and Joan Beaufort.[217] Their births were the foundation for the future Tudor dynasty through their descendant Margaret Beaufort. But before that, Katherine was married at the age of 15 to Hugh Swynford, and had two children with him, Blanche and Thomas. Katherine was a real-life heroine of courage, her six known pregnancies defying the dangers of medieval motherhood to begin a new dynasty, eschewing propriety in front of the judgmental eyes of England's medieval courtiers.

Hainaut in the 1350s was a bustling crossroads, its people were industrious and savvy, conducting business under a northern sky. In the 1350s, Katherine's father, Paon de Roet, was a knight of modest reputation, in service to Queen Philippa, the Hainaut-born wife of England's King Edward III, whose marriage tied their homeland to the English Crown. Katherine, probably born in a simple stone-walled manor near Mons, grew up in a household that had high standards. Her mother, whose identity remains unknown to history, raised Katherine alongside her siblings, and her elder sister, Philippa de Roet, would later marry Geoffrey Chaucer, a courtier and writer whose works are still read today. As a young girl, Katherine learned the usual domestic skills of a gently bred young lady – spinning flax, managing servants, and perhaps reading tales of chivalric valour. Around 1355, when Katherine was around 5 years of age, Sir Paon's service to Queen Philippa brought the family to England, thrusting them into the lively, multilingual world of Edward III's court at Westminster. The courtiers spoke French, Latin, and English, and its hallways were filled with knights, ladies, and envoys. Katherine adapted swiftly, and eventually her Hainaut accent faded away as she embraced her surroundings. Her father's loyalty to Queen Philippa and her sister's court connections would soon determine Katherine's future path.[218]

Jumping ahead to 1365, we find the 15-year-old Katherine married to Hugh Swynford, a Lincolnshire knight whose loyalty to John of Gaunt, Edward III's third son, tied him to the Plantagenet power structure. Sir Hugh's family held Kettlethorpe Manor, a modest estate of fields and forests. This marriage was arranged to strengthen Sir Paon's ties to John of Gaunt's retinue; it was a practical union but not without affection. Katherine settled into the life of a chatelaine – managing the manor's accounts, overseeing harvests, and learning the demands of a knight's household as she had been taught to do as a girl. Her first pregnancy came around 1366, when she was 16. Katherine, at Kettlethorpe, would have relied on local midwives, women skilled in herb craft and the art of helping women in labour.

Blanche Swynford, named for John of Gaunt's late wife Blanche of Lancaster, was born around 1366 at Kettlethorpe, in rooms warmed by a fire to counter the damp Lincolnshire air. The delivery was a private affair, attended by midwives and perhaps a trusted friend or sister, as was customary for a knight's wife. Medieval birthing practices emphasised a warm, enclosed environment, with the mother lying on a straw mattress supported by cushions or on a birthing stool. Midwives might have used warm cloths or herbal infusions to soothe Katherine, helping her cope with the challenges of labour, which could last from a few hours to a day or more. No records detail Blanche's birth, but her survival demonstrates a successful delivery. Katherine, young and healthy, would have recovered within the customary 30–40 days of 'lying-in', a period of rest to prevent postpartum complications. Blanche's birth improved Katherine's standing as a knight's wife. A healthy child was a sign of fertility and a promise of future heirs, critical in medieval society where profligacy secured social status.

Two years later, around 1368, Katherine entered into her second pregnancy at the age of 18. This time she had a baby boy – Thomas

Swynford, named for her husband Hugh's lineage. Thomas was born at Kettlethorpe, perhaps even in the same fire-lit chamber, attended by midwives who employed time-tested techniques like massage, herbal infusions and prayers to Saint Margaret or the Virgin Mary. The midwives would have monitored Katherine closely, using their experience to detect signs of distress, such as prolonged labour or excessive bleeding, which might require interventions like doses of shepherd's purse tincture for bleeding or repositioning the infant within the womb in order to shift him into a more favourable position. Thomas survived infancy, thanks to Katherine's careful postpartum care and the manor's relative isolation, which shielded her children from urban diseases like dysentery, smallpox, or plague, which infected England in waves. Raising Blanche, now 2, and newborn Thomas, Katherine learned how to balance motherhood with her manor duties, teaching her children basic letters and manners while managing crops and servants, her practical Hainaut education fortifying her with the skills necessary to protect their health in a world where childhood fevers were a constant threat.

Hugh's death in 1371, during a campaign in Aquitaine, left Katherine a widow at 21. Blanche, 5, and Thomas, 3, were now solely dependent on her, and Kettlethorpe's modest income offered them very little security. Widowhood in the fourteenth century equated vulnerability, but Katherine's resilience was formed in Hainaut's pragmatic ethos and she forged bravely onward. By 1372, she found a job as governess to John of Gaunt's daughters, Philippa and Elizabeth, in his vast household. John of Gaunt, at 32, was an impressive personage – Duke of Lancaster and lord of lands from Yorkshire to Bordeaux, he was a pillar of Edward III's reign. His first wife, Blanche, died of the dreaded plague in 1368, leaving three surviving children, and his 1371 marriage to Constance of Castile was a strictly political alliance for a Spanish infanta, devoid of affection. Katherine brought order to his household, helping his daughters with their lessons in Latin, music, and manners at Kenilworth's nursery. Katherine's steady presence was a welcome contrast to the court's chaos.[219]

The affair between Katherine and Gaunt began quietly, probably in 1372, in the glow of Lincoln's Great Hall, where copious amounts of wine and melodious lutes softened the court's formalities. Gaunt, overburdened from wars and politics, found in Katherine something novel – a partner who matched him in numerous ways. At 22, she understood the risks of loving a duke whose every move was scrutinised, especially as a widowed mother with young children. Their bond was passionate yet discreet, her governess role acting as a shield against outright scandal. By 1373, Katherine was pregnant again, her third childbirth at 23. She retreated to Kettlethorpe for the delivery, away from court scrutiny where the stigma of illegitimacy could not reach her and her children. The name Beaufort was chosen by John of Gaunt for his offspring by Katherine, after Beaufort Castle in Champagne, France, a possession of his.[220] Baby John was born around 1373 in a chamber prepared with care, clean linens, a cosy fire, and a birthing stool or mattress to aid in Katherine's labour. Midwives, possibly the same women who attended her earlier births, would be there to support her in labour and care for her and the baby after the birth. The delivery was private, with no recorded complications. John's survival was a triumph, his birth a new beginning in Katherine and Gaunt's relationship despite the shadow of illegitimacy.

Two years later, around 1375, Katherine, at 25, was now expecting her fourth child. Repeated childbirths would have taken a significant toll as medieval women didn't understand the risks of malnutrition, weakened bones, or infections like puerperal fever, which would inevitably become fatal within days. Henry Beaufort was born at Kettlethorpe, joining his brother John in a household carefully shielded from courtly gossip. The delivery probably followed a similar pattern: a fire-lit chamber, midwives dispensing herbal infusions, and the tense wait for the cry of a healthy baby. Labour could be gruelling, and midwives would use all of their knowledge to keep the process moving forward – like walking with the mother to encourage contractions or applying warm compresses to ease labour pain.

Henry was born healthy, his wellbeing a credit to Katherine's care in a rural setting that was less prone to urban diseases like plague, which killed thousands in the 1370s. The Beauforts' illegitimacy was a constant challenge, but Katherine ensured that their upbringing was similar to that of Gaunt's legitimate children, with tutors and resources funded by his generosity: money, furs, and land grants that eased her burdens as a mother of four.[221]

In 1377, at 27, Katherine was pregnant again, her fifth childbirth in just over a decade. Thomas Beaufort's birth at Kettlethorpe, would put Katherine's endurance to the test. No records detail Thomas's birth, but his survival was another successful delivery, with midwives present to monitor for signs of distress, in either mother or baby. Thomas was a sturdy boy who thrived, his birth further reinforcing Katherine's role as the mother of Gaunt's bloodline. The court's gossiping grew louder; her affair was an open secret, and clerics decried her sin, but Katherine pressed courageously on, her focus on her children's survival in an era where fevers or dysentery claimed many little lives.

By 1379, at 29, Katherine was pregnant for the sixth time, delivering Joan Beaufort, her only daughter with Gaunt. Joan's birth, again at Kettlethorpe, was a milestone, as girls were valued for strategic marriages in a world of alliances. The delivery, of course attended by midwives, involved the same rituals – herbal infusions such as motherwort or raspberry leaf, prayers to Saint Margaret, and a warm chamber to prevent chills. Labour with a sixth child could be risky because the uterus may not contract as effectively in grand multiparous women, as well as other dangers like postpartum bleeding or puerperal fever. Joan's survival was a relief, as infant mortality was always an omnipresent concern, and girls were needed for crucial dynastic ties. No historical records confirm stillbirths or children who died young for Katherine.

Raising six children was a monumental task in a time when childhood mortality was a constant threat. By her early thirties, Katherine split her time between Kettlethorpe and Gaunt's castles, ensuring her children's health through attentive care, probably using wet nurses for her infants (a common practice for noblewomen) and protecting them from urban plagues by raising them in the fresh rural air of Lincolnshire. The Beauforts, though illegitimate, were educated as well as their half-siblings, learning swordplay, religion, and courtly manners. John, in 1383, was 10 years old and loved sparring with toy swords and dreaming of knightly valour, his identical dark eyes marking him as Gaunt's own son. Henry, at age 8, pored over books, his piety and serious demeanour a perfect match for a future in the monastery. Thomas, at the age of 6, was a very active child, riding ponies and playing at combat with his brother, while Joan at 4, charmed everyone with her mother's grace and sweet countenance. Blanche and Thomas Swynford, now in their teens, were also thriving, their excellent education reflecting their mother's love and care for them. Katherine's child-rearing strategy was deliberate: bear children who could serve her lover's dynasty, raising them as nobles despite their illegitimate birth, their survival a testament to her vigilance in a perilous and disease-riddled era.[222]

By her late thirties, Katherine was a figure of stoic authority. The court's disapproval stung, but her noble lover's devotion was unwavering, his many gifts of money and land ensuring her and their children's comfort. Her children grew steadily: John, 15 by 1388, was in training for a future knighthood; Henry, 13, was eyeing the church; and Thomas, 11, showed talent as a budding warrior. Joan, age 9, was poised for a noble match. Blanche and Thomas Swynford, now in their late teens, were also advancing, their futures tied to Katherine's influence. Her successful reproductive strategy of six healthy children had reshaped her destiny, her children a bridge to Gaunt's dynasty. Socially, she walked on a tightrope, defying the Church's moral codes, yet holding respectability as a governess. Her chambers were her haven, where music and laughter drowned out the whispers of political plots, though clerics publicly castigated her. Her children were raised among the peerage, blurring the lines of legitimacy with an education just as good as that of their noble siblings.

By 1390, aged 40, Katherine stood near the peak of her influence. Gaunt's marriage to Constance was deteriorating and his wife's health was declining rapidly. His affair with Katherine – nearly two decades strong – was a mainstay of his life. Her six children, Blanche and Thomas Swynford, and the four Beauforts, were her legacy, all healthy and poised for greatness. Katherine could not yet foresee that she would soon marry John of Gaunt, be elevated to Duchess of Lancaster, or witness the 1396 legitimisation of their Beaufort children. When at last Katherine finally wed the widowed John of Gaunt in 1396, she landed not only her own place in history, but also the legal legitimacy of their four children; a pivotal step that would ultimately enable her descendants to claim the English throne.[223] Of all the women who loved kings, but wore no crown, none left a mark on England's future quite like Katherine Swynford. Through her, the transitory stain of illegitimacy became the root of royal inheritance. Few mistresses in history have shaped a dynasty, but Katherine birthed one into existence.

Bessie Blount and Henry FitzRoy

Bessie Blount made her first appearance on the stage that was the Tudor court at the tender age of 14 in 1513. She was a cousin of Lord Mountjoy, chamberlain to Queen Katherine of Aragon. Before she became one of Queen Katherine's ladies-in-waiting, she lived with her parents in a manor house in Shropshire. Bessie was the daughter of Sir John Blount, a loyal knight, and Katherine Peshall, whose family ties through Mountjoy meant that she had the right connections to place her daughter at court. By all accounts, Bessie was a pretty, blue-eyed blonde whose virtues included graceful dancing, singing and other 'goodly pasttimes'. Queen Katherine had learned from her mother to look away when the king took a mistress – her father, King Ferdinand was known for his many infidelities. So, she was not surprised when Henry took up with Bessie Blount – he had already had other transient mistresses at this point. Eventually the king would remove Bessie from court and ensconce her in a small house in Essex that he leased from St Lawrence Priory. Here the king could enjoy himself with his teenage mistress without the prying eyes of the court upon them.[224]

On 15 June 1519, Bessie gave birth to a healthy baby boy. King Henry was overjoyed and openly acknowledged his son, giving him the surname of FitzRoy ('son of the king' in Norman French). Henry felt exonerated, obviously HE couldn't be the problem in the lack of heirs male. The child survived infancy and so obviously Katherine, Henry's queen, was the problem. By 1519, Katherine had endured at least six pregnancies, but only one child, Princess Mary, born in 1516, survived. Her losses – two stillbirths in 1510 and 1514, three sons dead in infancy in 1511, 1513, and 1514, and a final stillbirth in 1518 – were public tragedies that deflated Henry's ego and caused him endless anxiety about the succession. Henry FitzRoy's survival offered a welcome contrast, his birth and survival proof that Henry could sire a male heir, proof of his virility in a court where the absence of a legitimate son threatened his dynastic stability. The court exploded with gossip, with courtiers snickering behind the queen's back that Bessie had delivered what Katherine could not, fuelling intense debates about the succession. Spanish envoys, loyal to Katherine, reported the event with indignation, viewing Henry FitzRoy's birth as a slight to her queenship, while English courtiers celebrated, seeing the boy as a potential safeguard for the Tudor line. The gossip amplified tensions between Katherine's Spanish allies clashing with Henry's supporters, who prioritised a male heir, even one born out of wedlock, to rule after him. Henry FitzRoy's acknowledgment was a direct response to Henry's dynastic fears, positioning him as a potential heir, despite his illegitimacy, in a court desperate for stability.

Henry's advisers were sharply divided on this boy's role in the succession, and their perspectives reflected the high stakes of the king's quest for a son to rule after him. Cardinal Wolsey, Henry's chief advisor and political strategist, saw Henry FitzRoy as a vital asset in a dynasty with no legitimate prince. Cardinal Wolsey was made godson to the baby, ensuring that he would be raised as a noble, with a household that mirrored a prince's, preparing him for a potential role as heir or regent. By 1525, at age 6, Henry elevated his son to Duke of Richmond and Somerset, titles that were equivalent to those of a legitimate prince, a bold move that displayed openly his ambition for the child to possibly rule one day. Wolsey's pragmatic approach viewed Henry FitzRoy's health and sex as a hedge against the uncertainty of Princess Mary, whose status as a female heir was precarious in a patriarchal monarchy where a prince was expected to succeed Henry. Thomas More, a devout Catholic and Henry's cherished adviser, took a more cautious stance, his moral convictions opposing the elevation of a bastard over a legitimate princess. Thomas More feared that prioritising young Fitzroy could spark rebellion among nobles or alienate Spain, a key ally, as Katherine's nephew, Emperor Charles V, held significant influence. Spanish ambassadors protested the boy's fancy titles, viewing them as an insult to Queen Katherine, their reports fuelling diplomatic tensions that could destabilise Henry's alliances. Some sources suggest Henry considered legitimising FitzRoy, a radical idea that alarmed even Henry's lap dog Wolsey, who feared provoking Spain further.[225]

Henry FitzRoy was raised away from his mother Bessie Blount, who had been married off to Gilbert Tailboys, and together the couple took up residence in Lincolnshire. Little Henry's education was placed in the trusted hands of his godfather, Cardinal Wolsey, and was tailored to prepare him for a potential role in the succession, whether as a king or a regent supporting a future ruler. By the age of 6, he was established at Sheriff Hutton Castle in Yorkshire, his household like a miniature court staffed with tutors, knights, and servants dedicated to his care and education. His schooling was princely in its rigour, reflecting Henry's hopes for a son who could rule England. FitzRoy studied languages including Latin, music, and religion – his lessons were balanced with physical training in swordplay, archery, and horsemanship, skills that were essential for a noble who might one day rule. His household was royally lavish, adorned with fine tapestries, silver plate, and a large staff rivalling that of other nobility, a testament to his dynastic importance in Henry's eyes. Henry visited occasionally, his pride evident in FitzRoy's copper locks and blue eyes – traits that mirrored his own and reinforced his significance as a possible heir. The Tudor court watched closely, with gossip swirling about his future role. Katherine's supporters rallied around Princess Mary, and they resented FitzRoy's prominence, their loyalty deepening the divide with Henry's faction, who saw FitzRoy as a fallback if no legitimate son emerged. FitzRoy's strong constitution and glowing good health were a constant reminder of the fragility of Katherine's lost sons, amplifying his status in Henry's plans for a male heir to rule after him.[226]

By 1527, at 8 years old, Fitzroy's role grew more prominent as Henry's obsession with a male heir intensified as his wife became past the age of childbearing. The king's efforts to secure the succession centred on FitzRoy, whose grand titles and princely education signalled his importance in King Henry's eyes. The court's gossip increased exponentially, with some speculating that FitzRoy could supplant Mary, whose gender limited her appeal in a patriarchal system that favoured male succession. Spanish envoys reported these rumours with alarm, urging Charles V to press Henry on Queen Katherine's behalf, fearing FitzRoy's elevation would undermine Princess Mary's claim. It's interesting to note that a society as patriarchal as Spain had no issue with women rulers – Queen Isabella was a respected figure in their time.

Cardinal Wolsey maintained FitzRoy's lavish household, his upbringing preparing the boy for a royal future. But Thomas More opined a more cautious approach, rooted in Catholic principles which warned of the risks of elevating a bastard. More's opinion mirrored the court's moral undercurrent and the fear that FitzRoy's prominence could destabilise the realm. Henry FitzRoy, unaware of these complex debates that swirled above his head, thrived, his surviving letters revealing a bright, dutiful boy eager to please his father. Now his education was expanded to include diplomacy and courtly etiquette, preparing him for a role that might include governing as regent or even king if Henry's plans for a legitimate heir faltered.[227]

In 1533, aged 14, FitzRoy married Mary Howard, daughter of the powerful Duke of Norfolk, a strategic match designed to bind him to an old noble family without outwardly challenging the legitimate succession. The marriage was not consummated due to the extreme youth of the bride and groom. FitzRoy and Mary Howard relocated to Baynard's Castle in London, where he continued his education, mastering the rudiments of statecraft. His charm and resemblance to Henry increased his stature in the eyes of the Tudor court, but soon only temporarily as Princess Elizabeth was named as successor to the throne. Gossip at court speculated about FitzRoy's future, with some envisioning him as a potential regent for the princess, others as a rival to her claim. Wolsey's demise in the fall of 1529 and the rise of Thomas Cromwell in the 1530s shifted alliances away from young FitzRoy as Anne Boleyn's progeny were to take precedence. Thomas Cromwell was less interested in FitzRoy's succession, his focus was instead on Elizabeth and the potential heirs who might follow her. Yet FitzRoy's prominence kept him central to the court, his very existence a reminder of the king's ability to father sons.[228]

By 1535, aged 16, Fitzroy's health began to weaken, with signs of a pulmonary illness, very similar to what his uncle Arthur suffered at around the same age. The court's attention was now focused on the drama around Anne Boleyn and Henry FitzRoy's star faded.

FitzRoy's life ended tragically in July 1536, at the age of only 17, from consumption, at St James's Palace in London. His death was a quiet devastation for Henry, whose dynastic hopes had rested briefly on this vibrant boy, seen as a potential ruler to carry the Tudor dynasty forward. No children survived him, his marriage to Mary Howard did not produce any heirs as it had never been consummated. The court mourned him, but FitzRoy's promise faded into memory like a candle snuffed out too soon. His death underscored the fragility of Henry's line, with no legitimate son yet born to rule after him. FitzRoy's life had been a fleeting answer to his father's desperation, his birth a rare triumph where Katherine's pregnancies had yielded only one surviving female child. The court's gossip mill contrasted his life with Katherine's many losses, advisers balancing dynastic needs with diplomatic concerns. These debates revolved around him for nearly two decades. Thomas Wolsey envisioned him as a potential king, while Thomas More cautioned against the high stakes of placing a bastard boy on the throne. FitzRoy's titles, from Duke of Richmond to Somerset, were a bold statement of Henry's hopes and dreams that this son might one day rule. His story remains a vivid thread in the Tudor tapestry, a testament to a king's obsession with a son to rule after him, a promise unfulfilled in the quest for a secure dynasty.

Mary Boleyn, Mistress of Two Kings

Many fans of Tudor history think of Bessie Blount as Henry's primary mistress, but Mary Boleyn had usurped this post when Bessie was married off and sent away to the countryside with her new husband. Often eclipsed by her sister Anne's dramatic rise and fall, Mary's story is one of fleeting royal favour, personal survival, and enduring mystery, particularly surrounding the births of her two children, Catherine and Henry Carey, and the question of their paternity.

Mary was born around 1499 or 1500 at Blickling Hall in Norfolk, the eldest child of Thomas Boleyn and Elizabeth Howard. The Boleyns were not yet the towering figures they would become, but Thomas's diplomatic skill and Elizabeth's noble Howard lineage positioned them as powerful players in the courtly game of royal favour. Mary's early years were shaped by the expectations of her family's aspirations, her education equipping her with skills in reading, writing, music, dancing, and needlework, along with French that would later serve her well.[229]

At about 15, Mary's world greatly expanded when she accompanied Princess Mary Tudor, Henry VIII's sister, to France in 1514 as a maid of honour for her marriage to King Louis XII. When Louis died shortly after the marriage, Mary Boleyn remained in France, serving Queen Claude under the young, lusty, and roguish King Francis I. Here, whispers of Mary's romantic entanglements began to circulate, with Francis later claiming she was 'a great whore, the most infamous of all'. Whether this was truth or boastful slander deliberately meant to needle the English is uncertain, but Mary's time in France, from 1514 to 1519, honed her understanding of courtly love and the role of sex appeal in court politics. This time abroad polished her charm, beauty and sex-appeal, qualities that would soon draw the attention of another king.[230]

Mary was recalled to England around 1519, perhaps to advance her family's prospects through marriage. Mary would now experience firsthand the competitive world of Henry VIII's court. On February 4, 1520, she married William Carey, a gentleman of the king's privy chamber and a man well-placed to elevate the Boleyns' status. The wedding, attended by Henry himself, showed his royal favour, and Carey's subsequent grants of land and offices reflected the family's growing influence. Yet it was Mary's own allure that would soon place her at the centre of Henry's attention. Around 1521 or 1522, as Henry's dalliance with Bessie Blount was concluded and Henry was on the prowl for a new, pretty plaything, Mary became his mistress. Unlike Anne, who would later hold out for marriage, Mary was a more pliant girl, her affair with the king conducted with relative discretion. Henry, then in his early thirties, was a charismatic and sexy figure – athletic, cultured, and insatiable in his desires. Mary, described as pretty and fair, was less sharp-witted than her sister and must have fit the mould of a royal mistress perfectly, her role undoubtedly facilitated by her husband's willingness to look the other way.

This would be a brief affair, lasting a year or two before Henry's attention shifted to her sister Anne Boleyn by 1525 or 1526. Mary's time as mistress was no more than a pleasant interlude and there is no record of her seeking to leverage her position for lasting power. Her compliance may have shielded her from the dangers that would later consume her sister, but it also left her vulnerable to the whims of a court that thrived on a diet of royal favour and betrayal. During this period, Mary gave birth to two children, whose paternity would spark centuries of debate. Catherine Carey, born around 1524, arrived at the height of Mary's affair with the king. The timing alone fuels speculation that Henry VIII could have been her father. Also, intriguing is William Carey's accumulation of royal grants during this period – was he rewarded, perhaps for his acquiescence to the king's interest in his wife? Henry's precedent of acknowledging his illegitimate son, Henry FitzRoy, born to Elizabeth Blount in 1519, shows he was not averse to claiming royal bastards, yet he never did so with Catherine. This could mean she was Carey's daughter, or that Henry chose not to acknowledge her for political reasons, especially as his marriage to Katherine of Aragon was faltering and he needed Spain's allegiance.

The case for Catherine's royal paternity is compelling but not conclusive. Her name might honour Katherine of Aragon, reflecting Mary's service in the queen's household, or it could be a family name, not necessarily a clue to her father's identity. No contemporary portraits confirm a physical resemblance to Henry VIII, and unlike Henry FitzRoy, whose birth wagged the court gossip's collective tongues, Catherine's arrival passed without recorded speculation. Two years later, on March 4, 1526, Mary gave birth to her son, Henry Carey, as her affair with the king was likely waning. The choice of the name Henry is intriguing, potentially a nod to the king or simply a common name in the Carey and Boleyn families. Like his sister, Henry Carey received no special recognition from the king, and his later life as a courtier and soldier was notable but not suggestive of royal blood. In my opinion the children were not Henry's due to the fact no woman sexually associated with Henry ever had two successful live births.

However, historians still speculate about the paternity of Catherine and Henry Carey since the Tudor court was secretive and there were no clear records. William Camden and other historians in the seventeenth century called Henry Carey 'reputedly' the king's son, although there is no primary evidence to back up these allegations. Henry VIII's refusal to acknowledge either child is notable because he was forthright about Henry FitzRoy. The political climate of the mid-1520s, when Henry was becoming more obsessed with Anne Boleyn and the question of who would succeed him, may have made him less willing to recognise his bastards in public. The Boleyn family's silence is also important. Mary and William Carey kept a low profile following the affair, which might mean that the children were Carey's or that the family decided to be discreet to avoid scandal. Modern historians still don't agree – some, like Alison Weir, say that Catherine's birth during the peak of the affair makes her a likely royal daughter, while Henry Carey's later birth makes his case weaker; others, like Eric Ives, believe that the speculation is not supported by contemporary evidence.[231]

William Carey died abruptly in June 1528 from the sweating sickness. Mary was now a widow with two young children and not much means to support them. The Boleyn family was now focused on Anne, who was on her way to becoming queen, and Mary's status as a past mistress didn't advance their cause. King Henry gave her a small income, which may have been a sign of goodwill, but her role at court became less important. Mary made a brave choice in 1534 that went against her family's plans – she secretly married William Stafford, a soldier with little money, in a love match that shocked the Boleyns. Anne, now queen, was reputedly furious with her sister and banished Mary from court. This move ironically saved Mary from the family's terrible fall in 1536, when Anne and their brother George were put to death for treason and adultery. Mary went back to a calmer life with Stafford, where she had at least one child and lived simply until she died in 1543.[232]

Catherine and Henry Carey, her children, grew up in relative obscurity. But subsequently, they did well with their cousin, Queen

Elizabeth I. Catherine married Sir Francis Knollys and became a trusted lady-in-waiting to the queen. Henry, on the other hand, became Baron Hunsdon and was a military leader and courtier. Their prominence throughout Elizabeth's reign has led to rumours that she thought they were her half-siblings, although she never said so in public, or in private that we know of. The question of who their father is is still an intriguing part of Mary's history. As it can never be fully solved, it shall remain so. Were Catherine and Henry William Carey's offspring? He was a faithful courtier who was showered with royal favours since his wife was mistress to the sovereign. Or were they the illegitimate bastards of a king who cared more about having a prince in the royal nursery than anything else? The truth is hidden in the Tudor court, where secrets were kept as securely as power itself.

Mary Boleyn's life, while not as well-documented as Anne's, shows that she was a strong woman who was able to handle the dangerous intrigues of love and power. This goes against her reputation as just a mistress. Her brief and discreet affair with Henry VIII put her at the centre of a turning point in English history. After the affair had run its course, and her husband passed away, she chose to marry for love, even at the expense of her own merits in the eyes of her family. This demonstrates a quiet, subtle strength that is quite different from her sister's dramatic path. Catherine and Henry Carey's births are surrounded by rumours, illustrating how unclear their legacy is. These children may have had royal blood or only the weight of a courtier's name. But Mary showed an ability to survive and protect her family in a century when women's choices were limited and their lives arranged largely out of their own hands. Mary Boleyn's story is not one of victory or defeat, but of gentle, quiet strength. It is the story of a woman who loved, lost, and lived on in the chronicles of a king's fleeting passion and a ruthless court's constant watchfulness.

Chapter 8

Birthing the Renaissance: Midwifery Practices and Customs Across Europe in the Sixteenth and Seventeenth Centuries

Midwifery in the sixteenth and seventeenth centuries had many commonalities; by and large it was a female only sphere with men at the periphery – mostly only priests and physicians. Midwives were women in nearly all cases, serving the mothers in their communities. These women were usually trained by other experienced practitioners of midwifery, and they were schooled in the use of herbs and other natural remedies for childbirth as well as healing in general. It was common for neighbours to ask for remedies for childhood illnesses such as sore throats, baby colic or headaches from midwives in the community. Community midwives varied from country to country in terms of their educational status and many were literate, such as in the lower European countries like Holland. In the emerging Dutch Republic, the profession of midwifery stood out for its early formalisation and adherence to a certain standard of practice. Midwives, or *vroedvrouwen*, were trained through structured apprenticeships under civic oversight, particularly in cities like Amsterdam, where they were salaried and available to the poor. Training for them included rudimentary anatomical instruction from physicians or surgeons, a very progressive feature for this time that enhanced midwives' ability to manage complications. Dutch midwives used printed guides created by the government for their edification. The Protestant Church regulated the profession post-Reformation, requiring proficiency in simplified baptismal rites but emphasising practical skills over religious duties. This conformity to certain regulated standards elevated midwives' status, making Holland a model for professionalisation, although rural midwives still relied on traditional apprenticeships.[233]

An interesting side note is that the texts used by European midwives were written by men; across Europe, midwives were indispensable as birth attendants, healers, and guardians of women's knowledge, but the sixteenth century marked the beginning of a shift toward medicalisation. Male physicians and barber-surgeons, equipped with university training, began to assert authority over childbirth, particularly in urban areas. In England, male-authored texts criticised midwives' lack of theoretical knowledge, while in France, barber-surgeons provided anatomical training that foreshadowed an insidious patriarchal takeover of childbirth. In the Holy Roman Empire, physicians supervised 'complex cases', and in Italy, midwives collaborated with male practitioners, a precursor to later tensions. In Spain, the Inquisition's focus on religious purity indirectly strengthened male oversight by limiting midwives' autonomy. Holland's formalised system delayed this trend, but even there, physicians began to encroach on 'complicated deliveries'. These early developments, though subtle, planted the seeds for the rise of male midwives (accoucheurs) in the seventeenth and eighteenth centuries, corrupting the female-centred tradition of midwifery.[234]

The Midwives of Spain

Before the 1492 expulsion, Jewish midwives *(parteras)* were integral to Spain's multicultural society, serving Jewish, Christian, and Muslim communities in urban centres and rural villages. Their training was similar to their Catholic counterparts (*comadronas*) in that it was mostly informal, relying on apprenticeships and communal knowledge networks because medical education was largely inaccessible to women. Young Jewish women learned their craft by assisting experienced *parteras* during deliveries, observing techniques such as the use of birthing aids like stools and appropriate usage of herbal medicine, and the management of normal births. These apprenticeships, often arranged within Jewish communities or families, were hands-on, allowing apprentices to master practical skills like positioning mothers for optimal deliveries, using olive oil for the perineum and addressing minor complications such as prolonged labour.[235]

Jewish medical traditions were informed by the famous Jewish physician and scholar Maimonides, and this distinguished *parteras* from their Christian counterparts. This rabbi had been the personal physician of Saladin and had a profound understanding of human anatomy and healing in a time when such knowledge was scarce. Maimonides' writings on health and diet, widely respected in Jewish communities, influenced midwives' practice by advising pregnant women on nutrition and rigorous cleanliness. For example, *parteras* might recommend avoiding or adding particular foods to promote foetal health, drawing on Jewish dietary laws that emphasised balance and purity. These practices, rooted in a holistic view of health, were completely unheard of in Christian societies. The midwives who dispensed this information to their clients gained reputations for their skill and discretion, making them sought after by both Jewish and Christian mothers. In cities like Toledo, where Jewish communities thrived, *parteras* often served mixed clientele, bridging cultural divides through their expertise.

Religious duties were a significant aspect of all midwives' training, as the Catholic Church required them to be proficient in emergency baptisms to ensure infant salvation. Jewish midwives, navigating a Christian-dominated society, were trained to perform these rituals to secure their licenses from ecclesiastical authorities. This training involved learning specific prayers and the use of holy water, though some *parteras* adapted these practices to be more sympathetic to Jewish sensibilities, performing baptisms only when necessary to avoid scrutiny. Their ability to operate within Christian frameworks while maintaining their Jewish identity reflects their adaptability and the pragmatic coexistence of religious communities in pre-expulsion Spain.[236]

Herbal knowledge was a cornerstone of Jewish midwifery, blending Jewish, Islamic, and Iberian traditions. *Parteras* used unique herbs discussed in Hebrew texts such as Black Cumin, which strengthens the womb, calms postpartum cramps and boosts milk production. Rue was used to stimulate weak labour pains and to promote postpartum recovery; it was a herb discussed in Kabbalistic texts for its effects on the womb. These remedies were often prepared according to recipes passed down through oral traditions or recorded in Hebrew medical writings, which circulated within Jewish communities. In Seville, Jewish midwives were known for their expertise in compounding herbal mixtures, a skill that enhanced their reputation as healers beyond childbirth. They also served as confidantes, advising women on reproductive health, fertility, and postpartum care, reinforcing their role as guardians of women's knowledge.

Socially, Jewish midwives held a respected but complex position. In urban areas like Granada, they served both elite and poorer families, and they were renowned for providing affordable care to marginalised communities. Their help was particularly valued in Jewish households, where they ensured ritual cleanliness and adherence to Jewish practices, such as handwashing – a practice unique to their society. Christian families also sought their services, drawn by their reputation for skill, cleanliness and confidentiality, particularly in cases of illegitimacy or sensitive births. This cross-cultural role positioned *parteras* as mediators in Spain's diverse society, though it also exposed them to scrutiny from Catholic authorities wary of Jewish influence.[237]

The absence of formal guild structures for midwives in Spain meant that *parteras* relied on community networks for professional legitimacy. Unlike in Italy, where midwives were regulated by guilds, Spanish midwives, including the Jewish ones, operated under ecclesiastical oversight, with licenses granted by bishops or local clergy. These licenses required testimonials of moral character and competence, often obtained through community endorsements. Jewish midwives navigated this system by demonstrating their adherence to Catholic baptismal requirements, though their Jewish identity made them vulnerable to accusations of insincerity or heresy, even before the expulsion.[238]

The Edict of Expulsion and Its Immediate Impact

The 1492 Edict of Expulsion, issued by the Catholic Monarchs Queen Isabella and King Ferdinand, wreaked havoc on Spain's Jewish midwives. All of Spain's Jewish population was ordered to convert to Christianity or leave the country. Many *parteras* chose conversion, becoming *conversas* so as to remain in Spain and continue their practice, while others fled to other regions like Portugal, North Africa, or the Ottoman Empire. Those who remained and chose to convert faced intense scrutiny from the Spanish Inquisition, the Order created by the monarchs to enforce religious observance among *conversos*. The loss of Jewish midwives was catastrophic for expectant mothers and their newborn infants, particularly in densely populated urban areas where these midwives had been practicing, delivering high numbers of babies.

Before the expulsion, Jewish midwives, healers, and physicians were critically needed in cities like Toledo, Seville, and Granada, where they made significant contributions to the population. The Jewish *parteras*' expertise in childbirth and women's health, combined with their affordability, made them a popular choice for pregnant mothers of all religions. The sudden expulsion of these practitioners had a devastating impact on maternal care because their Catholic counterparts lacked their intensive knowledge of herb craft and general medical knowledge. The remaining Christian midwives struggled to meet the demands of the high numbers of pregnant and labouring women. In rural areas, where midwives were few and far between, the impact was less pronounced, but in cities with higher populations, the loss of the highly skilled Jewish midwives was devastating, and their absence contributed to increased maternal and infant mortality rates, though precise data from the period is limited.

The Inquisition's focus intensified on Jewish midwives after 1492, because they were suspected of secretly practising Jewish rituals, a crime they called 'Judaizing'. The most common accusations were insufficient Catholic baptisms and performing Jewish postpartum purification rituals. Even using certain herbal remedies might be considered heretical if utilised by a Jewish midwife. In Granada, *conversa* midwives were accused of delaying baptisms and using Jewish 'incantations' during labour. These accusations sent innocent midwives to trials, imprisonments, torture, and executions. These arrests were often based on vague or fabricated evidence, a favourite modus operandi of the Inquisition's campaign to impose religious conformity. The fear of being arrested by the Inquisitors forced these midwives to adopt Catholic traditions, such as using religious relics like St Margaret's girdle or reciting Christian prayers instead of using proven Jewish remedies, as a way to avoid detection, though ultimately it diminished the effectiveness of their practice.

The social role of Jewish midwives also shifted post-expulsion. While Jewish midwives had once been respected for their knowledge, *conversas* now had to cope with suspicion from their Christian clients. The Christian women under the care of these midwives questioned their religious adherence, while ironically, *conversa* women were cautious about seeking their services because of the fear of being associated with anything Jewish. This erosion of trust limited the ability of *conversa* midwives to practice freely and effectively, as they attempted to maintain a precarious balance between using all of their knowledge and skills while avoiding Inquisitorial scrutiny. In some cases, *conversa* midwives withdrew from public practice, serving only certain tight knit *converso* communities, which further reduced access to their expertise.[239]

By the mid-sixteenth century, the Inquisition's relentless campaign had effectively eradicated Jewish midwifery in Spain. *Conversa* midwives who kept practising were constantly scrutinized, and even minor deviations from Catholic practices, like using a traditional Jewish remedy or failing to baptise a stillborn infant, could lead to accusations of heresy. The loss of these midwives had profound consequences for maternal care for the women of Spain. In Toledo the absence of skilled *parteras* left poorer communities dependent on less knowledgeable and experienced Christian midwives, whose training often only consisted of brief apprenticeships and limited herbal knowledge. This dearth of knowledge directly increased risks during childbirth, as the gentile midwives simply could not replicate the expertise of their Jewish predecessors.

Despite the Inquisition's relentless persecution, some Jewish traditions persisted in secret among *conversa* midwives. For example, postpartum cleansing rituals which were observed by Jewish law were conducted discreetly within *converso* households, and at great risk. These rituals, which emphasised hygiene and spiritual purification, had to be adapted to look like Catholic practices to evade detection. However, the Inquisition's oversight made these practices dangerous, and many conversa midwives abandoned them altogether in order to avoid suspicion. The loss of these traditions not only diminished the cultural richness of Jewish midwifery, but also reduced the holistic care that Jewish midwives had previously provided to their clients, which combined together both medical and spiritual practices.

The persecution of *conversa* midwives also affected the Catholic midwives, as the Inquisition's climate of fear discouraged the sharing of knowledge and information across the profession. Christians also faced accusations of heresy if they were caught using ‘unconventional’ remedies, so they too had to resort to the Church-approved practices, like prayers and relics over medical techniques. This shift effectively shut down the development of midwifery in Spain, as midwives gave up the use of certain herbs or ‘Jewish’ methods. The resulting constraints in training and regimen further compounded the loss of Jewish midwives’ knowledge and expertise, and the profession became increasingly standardised, allowing only the approved Catholic practices.

In locations that Jewish midwives escaped to, such as Portugal and North Africa, their skills enriched the local practices of the native midwives there. They brought their knowledge of childbirth and herbal remedies to new communities, contributing to birthing traditions in the Ottoman Empire or Moroccan Jewish communities. In Salonica, exiled Spanish-Jewish midwives adapted their practices to local customs, blending together the different traditions and their medical knowledge, with superior results. However, in Spain their absence left a void for expectant mothers, with the midwives that remained informally trained and heavily censored by the Church.[240]

The loss of skilled midwifery practitioners increased maternal and infant mortality rates, especially in urban centres where the demand for skilled midwives was high. Christian midwives, while numerous, lacked the same level of expertise, particularly in handling complications like breech births or postpartum haemorrhage. The social community of childbirth was also altered to deleterious effects. Jewish midwives had served as cultural intermediators, creating bridges of trust across religious and social boundaries. Their exile destroyed these networks, leaving the Catholic midwives to fend for themselves in a much more polarised society. The fear of the Inquisitors created a cautious approach to midwifery, with gentile midwives afraid to come under its scrutiny. In other regions, like Holland, where they incorporated rudimentary anatomical training, Spanish midwives remained restricted to the traditional superstition-based practices, mandated by Catholic religious oversight. [241]

The rise of male physicians in the late sixteenth century further marginalised midwives, as the seeds of medicalisation in the field of childbirth began to take root. Texts written by men and the increasing involvement of barber-surgeons in ‘complicated’ deliveries challenged midwives' authority, a trend that was made worse by the loss of knowledgeable, Jewish midwives. While male midwives (accoucheurs) would become more prominent in the seventeenth century, the sixteenth-century decline of *parteras* weakened the profession's foundation, making it more vulnerable to these shifts.[242]

The experience of Jewish midwives in pre- and post-expulsion Spain provides a window onto the complex ways in which gender, religion, and medicine were woven together in the social, cultural, and political climate of the sixteenth century. Before 1492, Jewish midwives were renowned for their skill and versatility, they served their communities as healers and cultural intermediaries. Their training was due in large part to the Jewish medical teachings of Maimonides along with practical childbirth experience. Maimonides built a system of healing based on the ideas of balance. He advocated for good, well-rounded nutrition, exercise and preventative medicine, revolutionary ideas for this time. The Jewish midwives were literate women who read the writings of Maimonides and these teachings allowed them to confidently address a wide range of maternal needs, from prenatal care to postpartum recovery. In big cities like Seville, these midwives were well liked for their discretion in cases of out-of-wedlock births, securing the trust of women in these communities.

The Inquisition's repression of Jewish midwives was devastating for Spain. Inquisition trials of midwives are documented, and they reveal how the *conversas* were forced to prove their adherence to Catholicism although even this often didn't save them from torture or death. Jewish midwives had to forgo their skills in the birthing chambers to have any hope of survival. The loss of these midwives not only reduced an expectant mother's access to skilled care but also eroded the cultural diversity of midwifery in Spain, because Jewish knowledge was replaced by Catholic rituals that had no efficacy.

In Granada, where *parteras* had served both Jewish and Christian families, their absence left these lower-income mothers with less skilled practitioners, and this switch increased their risks during childbirth. The psychological toll for pregnant or postpartum women was also significant, because the communal support that had been provided by

Jewish midwives was eliminated. The Inquisition's legacy reached beyond the immediate persecution of Jews; it re-shaped the social and medical landscape of childbirth in Spain.

Jewish midwives in pre-expulsion Spain had been vital to good maternal care; their skills had been learned through long years of apprenticeships as well as Jewish medical traditions. The 1492 expulsion and subsequent trials created a dearth of skilled care that Christian midwives could not fill. The loss of *parteras* not only increased risks for expectant mothers but also stifled the development of the profession of midwifery, because the fear of heresy curtailed its effectiveness. Jewish midwives found new positions within exiled communities, but in Spain, their demise was a turning point that highlights the profound impact of religious persecution on women's reproductive health.

Midwifery in the Emerging Netherlands

The midwifery profession during the sixteenth and seventeenth centuries in the newly emerging Netherlands was completely different from any place else in Europe, especially in Holland. Midwifery in this region was female-dominated, just as it was in other European countries. Midwifery evolved from an informal, apprentice-based practice into a standardised profession overseen by civic administrations. Midwives were known as *vroedvrouwen* (literally 'wise women'). Dutch midwives were set apart from their counterparts in other countries due to their structured training, access to rudimentary anatomical knowledge, and integration into municipal healthcare systems. In the sixteenth century, midwifery in the Netherlands had to adapt to the region's burgeoning urban culture. The profession became more regulated and science-based due in part to religious tolerance, even under Habsburg rule. Midwives were essential to community life, they were the primary birth attendants and women's health practitioners in both urban and rural settings.[243]

Training for *vroedvrouwen* in the sixteenth century still relied primarily on apprenticeships, a common practice shared by all midwives across Europe, but with civic oversight that was unique to the Dutch. Young women from mostly middle economic classes learned the trade by assisting experienced midwives at deliveries. These apprenticeships were frequently arranged through the government or medical guilds in cities like Amsterdam, where mentors were carefully selected for their reputation and skill. The process could last several years and the young apprentices learned extensive hands-on skills. In Leiden, midwifery apprentices were required to attend numerous deliveries under supervision before practicing independently – this ensured consistency and proficiency before these *vroedvrouwen* went out on their own to attend births.

Unlike most other countries, Dutch midwifery in the sixteenth century benefited from rudimentary anatomical training. In cities, midwives had access to lectures or demonstrations by physicians or barber-surgeons, particularly in Amsterdam, where the city's medical guild was very active. These seminars introduced the basic concepts of anatomy, such as the structure of the pelvis or foetal positioning, helping midwives to have a better understanding of complications like breech births. Although this training was not equivalent to a university medical education, this exposure to human anatomy shows the Netherlands' intellectual openness. Europeans who practiced the healing professions in the Netherlands were influenced by Andreas Vesalius, an anatomist who revolutionised medical knowledge. Midwives were allowed to watch dissections of female bodies to better understand childbirth anatomy, and these lessons enhanced their competence.

Municipal oversight in Amsterdam and Utrecht required midwives to get licensed, a process involving examinations or testimonials of competence and moral character. These licenses were granted by a panel of physicians, surgeons, or senior experienced midwives and a baseline of skill had to be demonstrated by applicants in order to receive a license. In Amsterdam, for instance, midwives were examined on their ability to manage normal deliveries and recognise when to summon help for complications, such as dystocia. Licensed midwives, known as *stadsvroedvrouwen* (city midwives), were appointed as public servants and as such received salaries, tax exemptions, and even pensions. This gave midwives additional status and incentivised high standards.

Religious oversight was also a reality for these women, particularly before the Dutch Reformation in the late sixteenth century. Under the Habsburgs, midwives knew how to perform emergency baptisms, a Catholic duty believed to ensure the infant's salvation. Their training had to include learning Catholic prayers and rituals and the use of holy water for baptising infants in cases of stillbirth or imminent death. As the Reformation spread, particularly after the 1570s, Protestants simplified these rituals; they became more focused on basic baptisms over formal Catholic rites. This shift reduced the religious burden on midwives so that they could focus on their skills, though they still remained accountable to Church authorities for their moral behaviour.

Dutch midwives in the sixteenth century used the same simple tools their European counterparts, did such as birthing stools and herbs. Birthing stools were common, but midwives knew to use minimal interference for the best outcomes. Their techniques emphasised non-invasive methods, allowing mothers to control their own births.

Midwives held a respected position in sixteenth-century Dutch society, particularly in urban areas, where their civic employment and training afforded them a higher status. They served a diverse clientele, from wealthy merchants to impoverished families. In cities, midwives were able to offer free services to poor women with funds supplied by municipal budgets. Beyond childbirth, *vroedvrouwen* were looked upon as healers – they advised women on reproductive health, fertility, and if called upon, they could testify in legal cases that involved pregnancy or infanticide. Midwives are trusted with the lives of newborn babies, and this trust that they earned often made them guardians of women's secrets, building trust within communities. Unlike the Holy Roman Empire, witchcraft accusations were rare in the Netherlands. Midwives were respected and they were able to practice without fear of persecution.

The Netherlands, even under Hapsburg rule, allowed midwives to ply their trade in a diverse society that included Catholics, Protestants, and even Jewish communities. Jewish midwives were less prominent than in pre-expulsion Spain, but they did serve their communities, even occasionally gentile women, bringing their own unique medical knowledge to bear. The spread of Protestantism in the late sixteenth century created a more practical and less religious aspect to midwifery, emphasising civic responsibility and service over religion. This environment supported midwives' professionalisation, as there was more concern for public health and maternal care than religious rituals.

The seventeenth century, often referred to as the Dutch Golden Age, advanced the profession of midwifery, as the newly independent Dutch Republic invested so much in public health and intellectual pursuits. Midwifery became increasingly formalised and uniform due to structured training programs, printed manuals, and better regulation. Dutch *vroedvrouwen* were arguably among the most professionalised midwives in Europe. By the seventeenth century, training for midwives in Holland had become an even more systematic process. Apprenticeships remained central, but they were now monitored by strict municipal regulations. In Amsterdam, apprentices trained under licensed experienced senior midwives – 'stadsvroedvrouwen' – for a minimum of two to three years. They were expected to attend a specified number of deliveries as an apprentice before applying for licensure. This formalised approach ensured that trainees gained comprehensive experience in managing normal births, recognising complications, and observing postpartum care.

The introduction of formal training programs in Amsterdam and Leiden vastly improved the profession of midwifery. By the mid-seventeenth century, Amsterdam had built a training school for midwives, one of the earliest in Europe, where trainees learned from experienced *vroedvrouwen* and physicians. These programs included lectures on anatomy, obstetrics, and pharmacology, taught by doctors in the city's medical guild. Midwives learned about the mechanics of labour, the role of the placenta, and how to use herbal remedies with greater precision. The student midwives also received the latest in contemporary medical texts. Human dissections became common, allowing student midwives to study female anatomy firsthand, a practice which helped their ability to understand complex cases like twins or malpresentations.

The literacy rate among Dutch midwives was higher than in any other European region; women read printed midwifery manuals and sat for exams. Civic regulation was required for the profession of midwifery which reinforced rigorous licensing requirements. In Utrecht, midwives had to pass written exams as well as oral exams; a panel of physicians, surgeons, and senior midwives tested their knowledge of anatomy, delivery techniques, and emergency procedures. Licensed midwives were appointed as public servants, and their civic responsibilities extended beyond private practice to include serving the poor and testifying in legal cases. In Rotterdam, *stadsvroedvrouwen* provided free care to impoverished mothers, funded by city taxes, and so ensuring equal access to skilled childbirth services for all.

The Dutch Reformed Church did continue to regulate midwives' moral conduct, however, expecting them to behave according to the Calvinist values of piety and sobriety. The Church's influence on training was minimal compared to the rest of Europe in the sixteenth century because local councils took primary responsibility for midwives' professional standards. Midwives still knew how to perform emergency baptisms, but this ritual was simplified under Protestantism, involving basic prayers rather than complicated Catholic rites. This helped midwives to focus more on their childbirth duties, with the emphasis on practical care and public welfare.

Seventeenth-century Dutch midwives continued to use birthing stools, linens, and herbal remedies, but their techniques became more refined due to anatomical knowledge and professional training. They used precise methods for manual repositioning of foetuses, such as external inversion in the case of a breech presentation. They used herbal mixtures with standardised recipes, such as fennel tea for inadequate lactation or ergot for postpartum haemorrhage, prepared for them by pharmacists. The introduction of instruments like forceps, introduced by male practitioners, were eschewed by midwives due to their association with surgical intervention. *Vroedvrouwen* preferred their tried and tested natural methods of managing childbirth.[244]

The social status of Dutch midwives was at its peak in the seventeenth century, particularly in urban areas, where their roles as public servants along with their excellent training made them respected public figures. They served a wide range of clients, from wealthy burghers to impoverished families, and city midwives could deliver hundreds of babies annually. Their roles expanded beyond the birthing chamber to include gynaecological care and advice regarding the remedies for menstrual disorders or infertility issues.

Midwives were beloved cultural figures and were shown in Dutch Golden Age art and literature as symbols of wisdom and care. Paintings by Judith Leyster portrayed midwives as women of renown. Unlike their contemporaries in the Holy Roman Empire, *Vroedvrouwen* practised with confidence, without fear of persecution. The Dutch Republic's intellectual climate due to advances in science, medicine, and publishing, had a direct influence on the profession of midwifery. The University of Leiden, a leading centre of medical education, trained physicians who collaborated with midwives, sharing knowledge through lectures or consultations. The Dutch Republic were at the cutting edge of public health care initiatives, and they treated midwives as the most important guardians of infant and maternal wellbeing. The presence of Jewish and other minority communities enriched *vroedvrouwen*, as midwives occasionally exchanged knowledge with Jewish or immigrant practitioners.

The Protestant Reformation which was solidified in the seventeenth century, changed midwifery by emphasising civic duty and practical service. Calvinist principles of discipline and community made skilled care a priority for all. This intellectual approach created an environment where midwives could thrive as both traditional healers and modern practitioners.[245]

Despite their advancements and possibly because of them, Dutch midwives faced challenges from the growing influence of male physicians and barber-surgeons. The late sixteenth century was the beginning of medicalisation of birth, as male practitioners began to supervise complicated deliveries. By the seventeenth century, this trend became more popular, with physicians like François Mauriceau publishing obstetrical texts that emphasised scientific authority over traditional knowledge. In Holland, midwives were able to maintain their autonomy due to their formalised training and civic support, but they were increasingly required to defer to physicians in cases of dystocia or other complications.[246]

The introduction of forceps by the Chamberlen family in England, though not widely adopted in the Netherlands until the eighteenth century, stirred up debates in the midwifery community over the role of instruments in childbirth. Dutch midwives resisted the use of forceps; they saw them as invasive and associated them with male practitioners who lacked practical experience in normal childbirth. This tension between female-centred midwifery and male-led obstetrics foreshadowed the rise of accoucheurs in the eighteenth century. Accoucheurs would soon challenge female midwives' dominance across Europe with disastrous results. Although Dutch midwives enjoyed a higher status than their counterparts in many regions, they had to submit to male physicians that were at the top of medical hierarchies. At this time, women were banned from receiving a university education, and this limited their access to more advanced knowledge. This lack of a university degree reinforced the perception that midwives were inferior to medical doctors. The encroachment of men into the previously female only sphere of childbirth was about to implode.[247]

Midwives in the Holy Roman Empire

In the Holy Roman Empire of the sixteenth and seventeenth centuries, midwives were indispensable, just as they were elsewhere in Europe. Unfortunately, the suspicious nature of this region constantly threatened the lives of these midwives with accusations of sorcery. The midwives faced relentless scrutiny from neighbours, civic authorities, and religious institutions. Their intimate role in childbirth made them essential yet feared; older women who used herb craft and dealt in the realms of birth and death were especially targeted by ignorant and fanatical peasants. The overseeing civic authorities imposed stringent regulations on midwives, and the Church governed their religious duties, marginalising midwives as outsiders despite their critical contributions.[248]

In a society gripped by religious fervour, poverty, and fear of the supernatural, midwives were seen with a volatile mix of necessity and suspicion. Every action a midwife took was scrutinised for signs of incompetence, immorality, or malevolence. This distrust was whipped into a frenzy by Lutheranism which made midwives scapegoats for all sorts of imaginary reasons. Midwives' contributions were tainted by the constant threat of accusations in rural villages and urban cities alike. On the outskirts of towns, such as in the villages of the Duchy of Württemberg, midwives were the sole guardians of childbirth, and their presence was critical for places where physicians were few and travel was hindered by rugged terrain, plague, or war. In a village like Urach in 1590, with its 500 inhabitants, a midwife's arrival at a birth was seen as a blessing and, quite literally, as a possible curse. The tools used by midwives such as swaddling cloths, a sharpened knife for cutting umbilical cords, vials of herbal oil, and various dried herbs were essential for the midwife, but was often a source of unease for the peasants. The labouring woman's family watched the midwife closely, fearing that her tools and remedies had the ability to bring harm or evil. Childbirth had inherent risks – infant mortality hovered between 25–30 per cent, and maternal deaths were always a possibility. The communal nature of childbirth compounded the dangerous nature of midwives' practice. Births were social events, bringing together female kin and neighbours to the birthing chamber. These gatherings sometimes became less a space of solidarity than a stage for surveillance, where a midwife's every action was watched with suspicion. A stillbirth, like the one recorded in a Swabian village in 1595, started rumours of a midwife's negligence – her neighbours whispering that her rosemary infusion might have been a deadly potion. Distrust stalked her every action.[249]

Suspicions like this were magnified by the very nature of birth – a moment fraught with peril in a spiritual sense as well as a literal one. In Lutheran Württemberg, midwives were expected to perform Nottaufen (emergency baptisms) for newborns at risk of death, reciting the precise formula: 'I baptise you in the name of the Father, the Son, and the Holy Spirit'.

One single error could incite community outrage. In 1610, in the rural village of Württemberg, a midwife hesitated during a baptism, causing the child's death to be unbaptised, and this led to the midwife being accused of spiritual negligence. The villagers shunned the midwife as a pariah, destroying her livelihood. The fear of the Wechselbalg, a demonic imp believed to replace healthy infants with sick ones, further intensified scrutiny for midwives. I suppose these child-switching devils had a particular love for unsuspecting midwives? I digress…

When neighbours watched the midwives dispense herbal remedies, they sometimes feared sorcery was involved. The witch-hunts of the period were particularly intense in German-speaking regions, where they viewed midwives as possible witches due to their role in life-and-death moments. This increased the isolation of these skilled women in a society primed to see evil in the profession of midwifery.[250]

In urban centres like Tübingen, a university town in Württemberg, midwives had to contend with formalised scrutiny that laid bare their utter lack of autonomy. The municipal council was motivated by their Lutheran concerns for 'order and population stability' amidst the Thirty Years' War, subjecting the midwives to stringent oversight through the Hebammenrat (midwifery board). This board was created in the late sixteenth century, and was comprised of the town clerk, senior midwives, and occasionally a university physician who enforced licensing. They required midwives to swear oaths to serve all women, report births to the civic registry, and avoid 'superstitious' practices. In 1615, Tübingen's records detail a midwife's examination, where she faced gruelling questions on managing breech births, treating postpartum haemorrhage, and performing Nottaufen. Her skills were in doubt until proven, and failure to obtain a license relegated her to the status of a Winkelfrau (corner woman). This reduced the midwife to the status of an unlicensed practitioner who would be shunned by authorities and distrusted by clients. Even senior licensed midwives were vulnerable; a 1624 inquiry into a midwife's handling of a postpartum fever case caused her to be summoned before the council, destroying her reputation and livelihood with spurious accusations of neglect, a stark reminder of her precarious position.

Religious fervour made the scrutiny of midwives more dangerous. In Lutheran Tübingen, the Church required midwives to ensure newborns' baptismal salvation, training them in Nottaufen and mandating reports of all births within twenty-four hours. A 1618 ordinance enforced this and pastors had to inspect the midwives' adherence to all religious protocols. In 1623, a midwife was questioned for mispronouncing the baptismal prayer and her error was turned into an accusation of deliberate spiritual negligence, which ruined her reputation. In Catholic Augsburg, Counter-Reformationists had similar oversight – the priests liked to test midwives on their knowledge of sacramental procedures, hoping to catch her out on any small mistake. In Rothenburg ob der Tauber, a 1605 case speaks of a midwife being questioned by the local pastor for forgetting to report a birth promptly. Her delay was interpreted as a disregard for Christian principles, putting her at risk of losing her profession in a community that held midwives to ridiculously high standards.[251]

Civic and religious oversight was compounded by community distrust, which permeated every aspect of a midwife's work. In Tübingen, midwives were expected to serve rich and poor alike, but their economic dependence on clients made them vulnerable. Wealthy families paid in cash: 12 kreuzer for a merchant's wife in 1622, while poorer ones offered goods like food, cloth, or eggs in trade for services. The midwives' birth records were inspected for 'overcharging', as seen in a 1620 fine for demanding payment from a labourer's family. Neighbours got wind of this information and used it to accuse midwives of favouring wealthy clients or neglecting the poor. In a 1619 Tübingen birth, some village women criticised a midwife for her use of a linen sling to support the mother's hips, questioning its necessity. Their petty complaints created unnecessary anxieties about the competence of the midwife in question. In rural Swabia, a 1612 case describes how a midwife got shunned for accepting a hen deemed 'too valuable'; her neighbours' accusations made her out to be greedy, causing her business to collapse.[252]

The birthing chamber was supposed to be a space for female autonomy, but it became a place where midwives could no longer feel safe in their profession. When women gathered to support the labouring mother, their presence also served to monitor the midwife, noting any deviation from expected practices. In Augsburg in 1600, a midwife's decision to reposition a mother during labour was debated by the women gathered there, their discussion escalating into a formal complaint made to the city council, accusing the midwife of endangering the mother. Male physicians from Tübingen's university began advocating for oversight of midwives in the late sixteenth century, citing their superior anatomical knowledge. This added yet another layer, suffocating supervision of midwives. A 1597 ordinance required midwives to consult physicians in complicated cases, subordinating their superior expertise to male authority. Doctors were now beginning to insert themselves in the birthing chambers, inferring that women were never as knowledgeable as a man educated in a university.[253]

In rural areas, the oversight of midwives was less formal but no less oppressive. The clergy carefully monitored them, relying on complaints by the villagers to enforce the accountability of midwives. In a 1595 Swabian case, a midwife was arrested after a stillbirth because she used a decoction of ergot to enhance uterine contractions, and this was seen as sign of witchcraft. The lack of licensing left rural midwives open to the community's ad hoc accusations, like the one seen in a 1605 Franconian case where a midwife faced a community inquest after a mother died giving birth. This happened when her neighbours' testimony described her as careless, despite her thirty years of experience delivering babies. The midwife had to end her practice and go into hiding. In 1613, a Swabian village midwife was shunned after a neighbour accused her of using a 'demonic charm – a knotted cloth for the mother to pull on during labour, and she was left completely isolated after the local pastor barred her from church.[254]

Despite their marginalisation, midwives in the Holy Roman Empire developed sophisticated practices through a rigorous apprenticeship system, although their training was monitored under the mantle of intense oversight and distrust. In the absence of formalised education, the midwives learned their craft through hands-on experience, honing their skills in the birthing chamber under the watchful eyes of community and authorities. This training may have been effective but the midwives chafed under the regulations that sought to suppress women's traditional knowledge and enforce conformity. The oversight sought to minimise midwives in a suspicious, patriarchal society. Midwives began training typically in their late teens, under a senior midwife. In Rothenburg ob der Tauber in 1590, an apprentice spent five years learning to palpate a mother's abdomen to assess the baby's position, prepare comfrey poultices for postpartum swelling, and recognise problems like a tangled umbilical cord and childbed fever. In Tübingen, the Hebammenrat required three years of apprenticeship before the midwife could receive licensing, and candidates were tested under intense inquiry. Also in Tübingen, midwives are described as using folding birthing chairs for their wealthier clients, utilising gravity to help with the delivery, or beds with linen slings for poor women. Their tools included a sharpened knife for the umbilical cord, goose grease for lubrication, and clay pots for boiling water. Herbal remedies such as chamomile tea for nerves, ergot to stimulate stronger contractions, and shepherd's purse for bleeding, were prepared under civic oversight to avoid witchcraft accusations. A 1619 Tübingen ordinance required midwives to submit herbal recipes for approval, and one midwife was fined for using an unlisted rosemary infusion. During labour, midwives coached mothers with rhythmic instructions – 'Breathe, push, rest' – but in complicated cases, such as a transverse foetal position, a physician consultation was required as mandated in a 1612 ordinance. In a 1619 case, a midwife's attempt to turn a mal-positioned baby was halted by a physician. The highly qualified midwife was dismissed, leaving her humiliated.

Postpartum care was critical but also heavily monitored. Midwives cleaned mothers with warm water and applied comfrey salves to soothe torn tissues, and they carefully watched mothers for signs of kindbettfieber (childbed fever). If a mother was experiencing low milk supply, the midwives used nettle tea to boost her milk production. In Tübingen, these activities were documented in ledgers overseen by the Hebammenrat; and in a 1621 case, a midwife was reprimand for failing to record a postpartum visit. A midwife was expected to perform spiritual duties too, and in provinces like Nottaufen in Tübingen, Catholic rites were strictly regulated. A 1623 Tübingen case described a midwife being fined for a baptismal error, and her mistake also required her to make a humiliating public apology. In Augsburg, a 1607 case records a midwife getting fined for omitting holy water in a baptism – as a result she was condemned as heretical.[255]

Obstetrical manuals like Eucharius Rösslin's *Der Swangern Frawen und Hebammen Roszgarten* (1513) were crucial in the instruction of urban midwives, particularly in Tübingen, where the Hebammenrat required a midwife to be familiar with such texts. A 1616 examination tested a candidate on female pelvic anatomy, and if she didn't know it well enough, her traditional knowledge would be dismissed if it deviated from the manual. Rural midwives were often illiterate and they relied on oral traditions, but their practices were heavily monitored by pastors and elders.[256]

The midwives of the Holy Roman Empire were essential but profoundly marginalised. Their practices were maligned by a fanatical environment of distrust and relentless scrutiny. In rural Württemberg, they were important but looked upon with trepidation, their work watched by neighbours fearing witchcraft. In Tübingen, Augsburg, and Rothenburg, civic and religious oversight was used to formalise their marginalisation, subjecting them to licenses, audits, and religious oversight. No other health practitioners had such odious restrictions. Midwives became the lightning rods for misogynistic distrust which, when combined with religious zealotry, would become the fuel for the burning of witches.

In the Holy Roman Empire of the sixteenth and seventeenth centuries, midwives were cast into a maelstrom of suspicion, their essential role in childbirth eclipsed by accusations of witchcraft that branded them as the malevolent agents of Satan. Amid the religious convulsions of the Reformation and Counter-Reformation, the chaos of the Thirty Years' War (1618–1648), and a pervasive culture of fear, midwives' practices were constantly looked at under a proverbial microscope. Their intimate work in the birthing chamber with its ramifications of life and death made them prime targets for all sorts of accusations: stillbirths, maternal deaths, and spiritual corruption through witchcraft. Neighbours, government agents, and religious clergy viewed their herbal remedies, prayers, and practice as potential evidence of satanic pacts, fanning the flames of the witch-hunts that swept through German-speaking territories.[257]

Midwives in the Holy Roman Empire were uniquely vulnerable to witchcraft accusations due to their role in the precarious act of childbirth, where unexplained tragedies could be attributed to malevolent intent. In an era with high infant mortality (25–30 per cent), midwives became scapegoats for the deaths of infants that defied the medical understanding of the time. In rural Ansbach, a Franconian margraviate, midwives were faced with accusations that stemmed from pervasive village superstitions. In a settlement like Feuchtwangen in 1586, with its 350 inhabitants, a midwife's presence at a birth was vital but perilous. When a newborn died hours after delivery, neighbours pointed to her actions – like administering herbs to ease labour pains as witchcraft, claiming it was a 'witch's poison'. A 1589 case recorded a midwife accused of causing a stillbirth after using a herbal infusion to stimulate sluggish contractions – her neighbours testified that the remedy was a 'demonic brew'. These accusations were sadly not uncommon during the cultural hysteria of the Wechselbalg (changeling), a demonic entity believed to replace healthy infants.[258]

In the urban province of Ulm, a Lutheran-free imperial city, midwives had to contend with accusations that were largely driven by community gossip and overly zealous clerical supervision. In 1604, a midwife was accused of witchcraft after a mother died during childbirth. The midwife had made the labouring woman a marjoram compress in order to reduce perineal swelling, and this was interpreted as a 'cursed salve' by the woman's neighbours. One accusation is described as beginning with rumours in Ulm's busy grain market, where the peasants gossiped about the midwife's 'strange' behaviour – working by dim candlelight and muttering prayers. The rumours ran wild until they escalated into a formal complaint to the city council. The authorities were anxious to maintain order during a difficult time of economic hardship and plague outbreaks; they investigated swiftly, fearing that the gossip centred around midwives could spark civil unrest. The midwife's herbal knowledge, once a well-respected and common community resource, was now used as evidence of witchcraft.

Religious anxieties fuelled witchcraft accusations in regions like Passau, a parish with well-known Counter-Reformation sympathies. Midwives were expected to perform emergency baptisms in order to ensure the newborn child's salvation; in 1610, a Passau midwife was accused of witchcraft after a newborn baby in her care died unbaptised. Her delay in performing the rite was interpreted as a deliberate act to condemn the child's soul to Satan. Religious officials, guided by the *Malleus Maleficarum* text (1486), saw midwives as potential heretics. Burning a sprig of rosemary to purify the air in the birthing chamber was enough to accuse a midwife of witchcraft. A 1615 case speaks of a midwife who was accused of causing a neonatal death after placing a blessed saint's medal under the mother's pillow, a practice deemed 'satanic' by the local priest, illustrating how virtually anything could trigger accusations.

Economic tensions were enough to spark witchcraft accusations. In rural locations like Ansbach, midwives would often rely on payments in goods – oats, eggs, or wool – from poor families, but these transactions might be viewed with suspicion. A 1591 case describes a midwife accused of witchcraft after accepting a basket of apples. Her neighbours claimed it was payment for a spell that caused a child's illness. In Ulm, a 1606 case refers to a midwife accused of 'bewitching' a newborn after requesting some extra rye for her payment in lieu of money. Her motives were thought to be evidence of greed and witchcraft. These accusations are examples of how midwives' precarious economic status made them vulnerable to community resentment, triggering witchcraft allegations.[259]

Social dynamics could also contribute to witchcraft accusations. In Eichstätt, a Catholic provincial town notorious for its witch-hunts, a 1597 case describes how a midwife was accused of witchcraft after an unfortunate series of stillbirths. Neighbours who were stressed over famine and religious tension, pointed to her frequent nighttime visits to birthing women as evidence of Satanic activity. The accusations escalated when one of the grieving mothers complained about thc midwife's strange smelling herbs, and other villagers recounted her 'eerie herbs and prayers'. A trial and subsequent burning ensued. This case illustrates how social unrest, combined with gendered biases, turned midwives into scapegoats for the communities that they served.[260]

Witchcraft trials in the Holy Roman Empire were formalised and extremely brutal. Midwives faced a legal system that presumed guilt and relied on various methods of torture in order to extract confessions. The *Constitutio Criminalis Carolina* (1532) was the Empire's criminal code, and it defined witchcraft as a capital crime. They allowed convictions on the basis of testimonies, confessions, and physical evidence. Midwives were frequent victims of these processes, and many were burned at the stake. In Eichstätt, under Prince-Bishop Johann Christoph von Westerstetten, midwives here faced the most ruthless trials. In 1598, a midwife was accused of causing a mother's death after she applied a poultice to staunch the mother's bleeding. The trial began with neighbours' testimony, with these so-called witnesses testifying that the midwife's 'peculiar' herbs and 'whispered chants' were proof of witchcraft. The Eichstätt court was guided by the *Malleus Maleficarum* or the 'Hammer of the Witches', a book which suggested torture as the preferred method for extracting confessions. The midwife was subjected to interrogation, during which the interrogator demanded the details of her herbal remedies and rituals. Under torture, she confessed to a pact with the devil, a coerced admission that led to her execution by burning. The court's records describe her 'confession' of causing the mother's death through a spell, a common outcome in Eichstätt, where over 400 witch executions occurred between 1590 and 1630.[261]

In Lutheran Ulm, witch trials there were less frenzied, but they nonetheless had equally devastating outcomes. In 1612, a midwife was accused of causing a stillbirth after using a yarrow infusion to stimulate sluggish contractions during a long labour. The trial began with a civic inquest, prompted by the neighbour's complaints about her 'suspicious' demeanour during the birth. The Ulm council summoned witnesses – female relatives who testified that the midwife had used a 'strange' prayer. The court had her herbs examined by a physician who subsequently testified that they were 'unnatural'. In this case, the midwife was not subjected to torture due to Ulm's relative restraint. She was merely banished rather than executed, but her livelihood was destroyed and her reputation as a witch cemented in the memory of the community.

In the Catholic province of Passau, their ecclesiastical courts were central to witchcraft trials. In 1617, a midwife was accused of causing a baby's death after using a lavender salve. The trial was carried out by the Catholic court, beginning with a testimony from the mother's family, who claimed the midwife's 'secretive' behaviour – working by moonlight – implied she was using witchcraft. The court interrogated her on how she conducted baptisms on newborns, suspecting she had sabotaged the infant's soul. After the midwife was tortured with thumbscrews, she confessed to 'consorting with demons'. This forced confession led to her execution in 1618. The court's records highlight her 'diabolical' salve, exemplifying the Church's fear of midwives as spiritual threats.[262]

The social dynamics of witchcraft accusations against midwives gained its foothold in the fanatical and deeply misogynistic culture in The Holy Roman Empire of the sixteenth century. Midwives were professional women working outside male authority and thus were inherently suspect in a patriarchal society. Their oral knowledge of herbs and customs were passed down through the generations and within the male-dominated medical and religious establishments they were viewed with suspicion and fear.

In Eichstätt, the community's anxiety over economic hardships fuelled widespread witchcraft accusations. In 1601, a midwife was accused of witchcraft after a series of infant deaths in a village. Neighbours facing famine, starvation and conflict accused the midwife of witchcraft due to her frequent visits and use of unusual herbs. Gossip and the testimony of a grieving father fuelled the suspicion, leading to her trial and execution in 1602. This event had the effect of mistrust toward other midwives in the region. In 1615, a midwife was accused of causing a new mother's death after giving her fennel tea. Male physicians, asserting their anatomical expertise from texts like Vesalius's *De humani corporis fabrica* (1543), testified that her remedy was 'unnatural', aligning with the *Malleus Maleficarum's* view of midwives as witches. The trial, driven by the city council's desire to assert control, had the midwife banished, her expertise dismissed as sorcery. This case reflects midwives' marginal status as women, which made them vulnerable, and relegated their knowledge as inferior and a threat to male authority. The *Malleus Maleficarum* portrayed midwives as particularly prone to witchcraft, claiming that they killed newborns or offered them as a sacrifice to Satan. This stereotype helped to create a climate where midwives were presumed guilty before any evidence was even examined. In Eichstätt, the bishop's court targeted midwives as part of a broader campaign, with over sixty per cent of accused witches being women in healing roles. In Passau, Catholic records from 1610–1620 show midwives comprising twenty per cent of witchcraft trials, despite being a small fraction of the population. The Thirty Years' War also caused an increase in witchcraft accusations; contributing factors were the social and economic instability which heightened communal anxieties.[263]

Torture was often the modus operendi used to extract confessions from midwives. Thumbscrews, the Rack and the nail studded Iron Maiden were all employed in the torture of suspected witches in the sixteenth century. In Eichstätt, the strappado and leg screws were common, forcing midwives to confess to demonic pacts. In Ulm, where torture was less common, psychological pressure was brought to bear, such as prolonged imprisonment and starvation in order to force women to confess to witchcraft.[264]

Witchcraft trials had a devastating impact on midwives, shattering their livelihoods, reputations, and destroying their lives. In Eichstätt, executions deterred women from becoming midwives, leaving the women in this community alone in childbirth – putting the lives of mothers and infants at risk. In Ulm, banishments forced midwives to relocate, taking their life-saving knowledge with them. No midwives were open to serving in Passau after the executions of midwives became widespread, prompting them to abandon their traditional roles. In Ansbach, fines and restrictions served to isolate midwives, making their social and economic marginalization complete.

Witchcraft trials also reinforced gendered hierarchies. Branding midwives' knowledge as witchcraft empowered male physicians who began to overtake childbirth from women. A 1619 Passau ordinance required midwives to consult with physicians, thus placing their expertise into question. This shift marginalised female healers and childbirth became an increasingly male-dominated domain.

Midwives in the Holy Roman Empire were frequently accused of witchcraft due to their involvement in childbirth. In cities like Ansbach and Ulm, they faced allegations of causing harm through supposed sorcery, with trials driven by fear and legal procedures like the *Constitutio Criminalis Carolina* often relying on torture. Many midwives suffered execution, banishment, or fines, leading to their marginalisation.

Conclusion

Recorded history does not often begin with a woman in childbirth. There are few accounts of the anguished cries of a mother confronted with a child born dead. History is full of kings and conquests, bloody executions and bold treaties. We read the names of royal heirs, but the names of the midwives who delivered them are missing. Behind every crown and crisis of succession was a woman's womb, bleeding, contracting, waiting or mourning. In writing this book I sought to re-orient the reader's focus away from the glamour of the throne and on the triumphant – or anguished cries within the birthing chamber and the mothers and midwives within. What emerged inside these chapters is not just medical or political history, it is a visceral history. These are the missing stories of queens who suffered from countless lost children, children they had plans and dreams for. This conclusion weaves these stories together, not as isolated case studies, but as threads in a single painful tapestry.

We began with Margaret Beaufort, a teenage bride who created a dynasty through her act of giving birth. Margaret changed the face of England by merging together two warring factions and uniting them in peace through marriage. From there, we followed a succession of Tudor queens whose wombs were prized, prodded, doubted, and dissected in spite of the fact that no scalpel was ever placed upon them. In the case of Katherine of Aragon, we saw how the weight of expectations over nearly two decades destroyed her. She conceived repeatedly with most of her pregnancies ending in miscarriage, stillbirth, or in the death of her newborn child. Her faith, her sense of self, and ultimately her crown was tied to her inability to bear a living son, an heir to the throne for her husband and king. In Katherine's story we saw how the tragic fusion of fertility and legitimacy could rent asunder a family and a dynasty because political alliances hinged on something as unpredictable as the contraction of a uterus.

Anne Boleyn's womanhood had a more complex and paradoxical position within the Tudor court. Her quick conception with Elizabeth was a welcome symbol of hope for the succession but at the same time, a source of anxiety for her family, her court and her subjects. Elizabeth was the unwanted girl who would eventually become one of England's most iconic monarchs. After the initial disappointment of the girl's birth, her parents prayed for more children, more heirs – preferably boys. The fact that Elizabeth was a princess was perceived by many, including Henry VIII himself, as a disappointment in the dynastic struggle for a prince. This tension placed Anne's womb at the centre of the risky game of Tudor reproductive strategy which would ultimately never be won.

Following Elizabeth's birth, Anne endured a series of devastating miscarriages, and the one after Henry's jousting accident in 1536 would prove to be especially unlucky for Anne. These tragic losses were viewed through a myopic lens distorted by gender politics and court intrigue. In Tudor England, miscarriages were considered bad omens that heightened superstitions about divine displeasure and female inadequacy – especially when involving an unpopular queen like Anne. Her repeated miscarriages worsened her already fragile position, increased court anxiety, and indirectly damaged her reputation during her trial by reinforcing negative views and fuelling her adversaries' narrative. Anne was a failure as a queen according to the standards of the day. She began her tenure as queen as an unpopular choice in the views of many; and the lack of a surviving son was weaponised against her through rumours and gossip. Her body was scrutinised and politicised in ways which exemplified the anxieties over the succession and the unique role of queens in procuring dynastic continuity. A uterus became a contested space with political ramifications instead of a woman's private sphere. Anne's story demonstrates how a woman's capacity for procreation was used as a political tool, wielded and contested within the highest echelons of power. Her story highlights the perilous convergence of gender, politics, and physical autonomy in an era when a woman's value was tied to her ability to bear sons, and failure to do so could lead to ruin.

Jane Seymour, Henry VIII's third wife, had the unique privilege of producing the longed-for heir. Her body, after finally producing the much anticipated prince, sadly succumbed to a tragic and lonely death. Her singular triumph of childbirth cost her her life. In this moment, the king and his realm had what it wanted, a prince! Sadly however, the price was a queen's corpse. The silence around the circumstances of Jane's death reveal just how maternal mortality was so normalised that royal death in childbed was merely a footnote in the path to succession.

Where in all this drama was the midwives? Often overlooked are the quiet attendants of history's most celebrated births. In every childbirth chamber, a midwife was there to encourage the mother in her time of travail. They delivered the prince and the pauper alike with skilful, gentle hands. Midwives were the anonymous keepers of many secrets within the royal birthing chambers. This book is a testament to their rituals, their oaths, and their restricted, often feared power in the long shadow of The Church and Crown.

Delving into the depths of Kell-positive blood types, genetic disorders and conditions like McLeod's syndrome, we re-examined the biological realities that shaped the Tudor monarchy. Through these insights we can see how these were not simply unlucky women or victims of divine judgment, these queens were ensnared in the terrible web of hereditary blood incompatibilities. This is a science that was completely foreign to the sixteenth-century's medical compendium, but tragically it was a genetic reality that formed the Tudors' reproductive histories. What was once thought of as a curse or a divine punishment can now be understood as genetic fate. Still, even today, many women are made to feel that their reproductive losses are personal failures.

In the last chapter, we expanded our discussion of sixteenth-century midwifery to other European countries. Although the mechanism of childbirth was and is universal, the practice of midwifery certainly was not. The midwives of Holland enjoyed positions of respect and civil servitude and were able to receive excellent educations unique to women in this period. In stark contrast, the midwives of The Holy Roman Empire were seen through the lens of superstition, religious fanaticism merging with misogyny. Likewise, the midwives of post-expulsion Spain were subject to the mandates of the Inquisition and most of the well-educated

Jewish midwives were expelled. The common theme is the overarching patriarchal control that Christianity maintained over women, especially midwives whose female-centred sphere was uniquely challenging to both Catholicism and Lutheranism alike.

In this book, I have given readers a singular history of the intimate and misunderstood world of sixteenth-century midwifery. Travelling across the wombs of Europe, this book renumerates what history has neglected to record. In the anguished moans of Katherine of Aragon, the panicked cries of Anne Boleyn, the lonely weeping of Jane Seymour, and in the clandestine prayers of the Jewish midwives, this book gives a voice to their forgotten histories. One question remains – will history repeat itself? What happens when the womb cannot do what has been asked of it? Will women still be blamed, shamed and silenced in the dicey game of reproductive strategy?

As long as there are women willing to do the difficult but holy work of midwifery, women will have the solace of experienced and gentle care. I dedicate this book to every midwife whose hands have carried the weight of both life and death; and to every reader who has questioned the silence around reproductive suffering. I hope you can be reminded: the womb is not cursed, the silence around it is.

References

Introduction

1. Cressy, David, *Birth, Marriage and Death: Ritual, Religion and the Life-Cycle in Tudor and Stuart England* (Oxford University Press, 1997).
2. Ibid.

PART ONE

Chapter 1

3. Tallis, Nicola, *Uncrowned Queen: The Life of Margaret Beaufort, Mother of The Tudors* (Basic Books, 2020).
4. Halsted, Caroline, *Margaret Beaufort, Countess of Richmond and Derby. Mother of King Henry Vll and Foundress of Christs and Saint John's College* (Oxford, Smith, Elder And Co. Cornhill, 1845).
5. Ibid.
6. Ibid.
7. Tallis, *Uncrowned Queen.*
8. Garnica-Rosas, L., Maguiña, J. L., Arroyo-Acevedo, J. L., Rojas, K. D., & Herrera-Añazco, P., 'Determinants of adolescent pregnancy in indigenous communities from the Peruvian central jungle: a case–control study', *Reproductive Health*, 18(1), 202, p. 203. doi: 10.1186/s12978-021-01244-2.
9. Halsted, *Margaret Beaufort.*
10. Tallis, *Uncrowned Queen.*

11. Norton, Elizabeth, *Margaret Beaufort: Mother of the Tudor Dynasty* (Amberley Publishing, 2010).
12. Maltz, Wendy, *The Sexually Healing Journey: A Guide For Survivors of Sexual Abuse*, (William Morrow Paperbacks, 2012).
13. Tallis *Uncrowned Queen.*
14. Ibid.
15. Norton, *Margaret Beaufort.*
16. Ibid.
17. Tallis *Uncrowned Queen.*
18. Norton, *Margaret Beaufort.*
19. Tallis, *Uncrowned Queen.*

Chapter 2

20. Licence, Amy, *In Bed With The Tudors* (Amberley Publishing, 2012).
21. Ibid.
22. Ibid.
23. Cressy, *Birth, Marriage and Death.*
24. Loudon, I., 'Deaths in Childbed From the Eighteenth Century to 1935', *Medical History*, 1986; January 30.
25. Cressy, *Birth, Marriage and Death.*
26. Rösslin, Eucharius, *The Byrth of Mankynde, Otherwise Named the Woman's Booke* (1540).
27. Cressy, *Birth, Marriage and Death.*
28. Licence, *In Bed With The Tudors.*
29. Cressy, *Birth, Marriage and Death.*
30. Letters and Papers, Foreign and Domestic of the Reign of Henry VIII.
31. Cressy, *Birth, Marriage and Death.*
32. Ibid.
33. Ibid.

Chapter 3

34. License, Amy, *Elizabeth of York* (Amberley Publishing, 2013).
35. Ibid.
36. Weir, Alison, *Elizabeth of York: A Tudor Queen and Her World* (Ballantine Books, December 2013).

37. License, *Elizabeth of York.*
38. Weir, *Elizabeth of York.*

Chapter 4

39. Tremlett, Giles, *Catherine of Aragon: The Spanish Queen of Henry VIII* (Faber and Faber, 2010).
40. The Freelance History Writer, June 19, 2015.
41. Ibid.
42. Starkey, David, *Six Queens* (Harper Collins, 2004).
43. Letters and Papers Foreign and Domestic, Henry VIII, Vol. 12, Part 2.
44. Dewhurst, J., 'The Alleged Miscarriages of Catherine of Aragon and Anne Boleyn', *Medical History* 28(1), January 1984
45. Bideau, A., Desjardins, B. & Héctor Pérez-Bringoli (eds.) *Infant and Child Mortality in the Past* (Oxford University Press, 1998).
46. Chamberlain, F. *The Private Character of Henry VIII* (Vanguard Press, 1931).
47. Ibid.
48. Ibid.

Chapter 5

49. Starkey, *Six Queens.*
50. Ives, Eric, *The Life and Death of Anne Boleyn* (Blackwell Publishing, 2005).
51. Ibid.
52. Starkey, *Six Queens.*
53. Ives, *The Life and Death of Anne Boleyn.*
54. Ibid.
55. Starkey, *Six Queens.*
56. License, Amy, *Anne Boleyn: Adultery, Heresy, Desire* (Amberley Publishing, 2017).
57. Ibid.
58. Ibid.
59. Ibid.
60. Ibid.
61. Ibid.

62. Ibid.
63. Ives, *The Life and Death of Anne Boleyn.*
64. License, *Anne Boleyn.*
65. Ives, *The Life and Death of Anne Boleyn.*
66. Letters and Papers, Foreign and Domestic of the Reign of Henry VIII
67. Ibid.

Chapter 6

68. Gross, Pamela M., *Jane the Quene, Third Consort of King Henry VIII* (Edwin Mellen Press, 1999).
69. Ibid.
70. Ibid.
71. Starkey, *Six Queens.*
72. Ibid.
73. Whitelock, Anna, *Princess, Bastard, Queen* (Random House, 2009).
74. Starkey, *Six Queens.*
75. Letters and Papers Foreign and Domestic, Henry VIII, Vol. 12, Part 2.
76. Starkey, *Six Queens.*
77. Ibid.
78. Letters and Papers Foreign and Domestic, Henry VIII, Vol. 12, Part 2.
79. Gross, *Jane the Quene.*
80. Letters and Papers Foreign and Domestic, Henry VIII Vol. 12, Part 2.
81. Ibid.
82. Wriothesley, Charles, *A Chronicle of England During the Reigns of The Tudors From 1485 to 1559,* Volume 1, William Douglas Hamilton (ed.) (Forgotten Books, 2018).
83. Ibid.
84. Letters and Papers Foreign and Domestic, Henry VIII, Vol. 12, Part 2.
85. Ibid.
86. Ibid.
87. Ibid.
88. Ibid.
89. Ibid.

90. Wriothesley, *A Chronicle of England.*
91. Ibid.
92. Letters and Papers Foreign and Domestic, Henry VIII, Vol. 12, Part 2.
93. Wriothesley, *A Chronicle of England.*
94. Letters and Papers Foreign and Domestic, Henry VIII, Vol. 12, Part 2.
95. Wriothesley, *A Chronicle of England.*
96. Rösslin, Eucharius, *The Byrth of Mankynde.*
97. Wriothesley, *A Chronicle of England.*
98. Ibid.
99. Rösslin, Eucharius, *The Byrth of Mankynde.*
100. Wriothesley, *A Chronicle of England.*
101. Ibid.
102. Ibid.

PART TWO

Chapter 1

103. Dawkins, Richard, *The Selfish Gene* (Oxford University Press 1976).
104. Whitley, C. B., & Kramer, K., 'A new explanation for the reproductive woes and midlife decline of Henry VIII', *The Historical Journal* 53(4), pp, 827–848. (Cambridge University Press, 2010.)
105. Stride, P., & Lopes Floro, K., 'Henry VIII, McLeod syndrome and Jacquetta's curse', *Journal of the Royal College of Physicians of Edinburgh*, 43(4), pp. 353–367. (Royal College of Physicians of Edinburgh, 2013.)
106. Jayasena, C. N., & Shrimplin, V., 'Was Henry VIII infertile? Miscarriages and male infertility in Tudor England', *The Journal of Interdisciplinary History*, 52(2), pp. 155–176. (MIT Press, 2021.)
107. Whitley, C. B., & Kramer, K., 'A new explanation for the reproductive woes and midlife decline of Henry VIII', *The Historical Journal* 53(4), pp, 827–848. (Cambridge University Press, 2010.)

108. Wheatcroft, A., *The Habsburgs: Embodying Empire* (Penguin Books, 1995).

Chapter 2

109. Kramer, Cornelius Kyra, *Blood Will Tell, A Medical Explanation of the Tyranny of Henry VIII* (Ashwood Press, 2012).
110. Ibid.
111. Ibid.
112. Ibid.
113. Ibid.
114. Kramer, Cornelius Kyra, *Interpreting the Death of Edward VI: The Life and Mysterious Demise of the Last Tudor King* (Pen and Sword History, 2022).
115. Borman, Tracy, *Anne Boleyn & Elizabeth I: The Mother and Daughter Who Forever Changed British History* (Atlantic Monthly Press, 2023).
116. Doran, Susan, *Elizabeth I and Her Circle* (Oxford University Press, 2015).
117. Levin, Carole. *The Heart and Stomach of a King: Elizabeth I and the Politics of Sex and Power* (University of Pennsylvania Press, 2013).
118. Starkey, David, *Elizabeth: The Struggle for the Throne* (HarperCollins, 2001).
119. Ibid.
120. Skidmore, Chris, *Death and the Virgin Elizabeth, Dudley and the Mysterious Fate of Amy Robsart* (Phoenix, Orion Books Ltd, 2010).
121. Levin, *The Heart and Stomach of a King.*

Chapter 3

122. Rady, Martin, *The Hapsburgs: to Rule the World* (Basic Books, 2020).
123. Kann, Robert A., *A History of the Hapsburg Empire, 1526–1918* (University of California Press, 1974).
124. Stollberg-Rilinger, Barbara, *Maria Theresa: The Hapsburg Empress in her Time* (Princeton University Press, 2022).
125. Ibid.

126. Judson, Pieter M., *The Hapsburg Empire: A New History* (Belknap Press of Harvard University Press, 2016).
127. Winder, Dimon, *Danubia: A Personal History of Hapsburg Europe* (Farr, Strauss and Giroux, 2014).
128. Kann, Robert A., *A History of the Hapsburg Empire, 1526–1918* (University of California Press, 1980).
129. Stollberg-Rilinger, *Maria Theresa.*
130. Wheatcroft, A., *The Habsburgs: Embodying Empire* (Penguin Books, 1995).

Chapter 4

131. Clegg, Melanie, *Margaret Tudor: The Life of Henry VIII's Sister* (Pen and Sword History, 2018).
132. Watkins, Sarah-Beth, *Margaret Tudor, Queen of Scots* (Chronos Books, 2017).
133. Chapman, Hester W., *Margaret Tudor, Queen of Scots*, (Jonathan Cape, 1981).
134. Pitscottie, Lindsay, R., *The Historie and Cronicles of Scotland*, A. J. G. McKay (ed.) (Scottish Text Societie).
135. Watkins, *Margaret Tudor.*
136. Letters and Papers, Henry VIII, Vol. 1–4, 1509–1515.
137. Accounts of The Lord High Treasurer of Scotland, Vol. II, Thomas Fickson (ed.) (Edinburgh).
138. Letters and Papers, Henry VIII, Vol. 1–4, 1509–1515.
139. Ibid.
140. Ibid.
141. Ibid.
142. Chapman, Hester W., *Margaret Tudor, Queen of Scots* (Jonathan Cape, 1981).
143. Perry, Maria, *The Sisters of Henry VIII: The Tumultuous Lives of Margaret of Scotland and Mary, Queen of France,* (Da Capo Press, 1998).

Chapter 5

144. Loades, David, *Mary Tudor: A Life* (Basil Blackwell, 1989).
145. Porter, Linda, *The First Queen* (Piatkus Books, 2007).

146. Thomas, Melita, *The King's Pearl: Henry VIII and His Daughter Mary* (Amberley Publishing, 2017).
147. Whitelock, *Princess, Bastard, Queen.*
148. Calendar of State Papers, Spanish, Vol. IV, XI–XIII (1879–1954).
149. Porter, *The First Queen.*
150. Calendar of State Papers, Venetian, Vol. V–VI (1873–1884).
151. Letters and Papers, Foreign and Domestic, of the Reign of Henry VIII, Vol. VI, XXI (1882–1920).
152. Edwards, John, *Mary I: England's Catholic Queen* (Yale University Press, 2011).
153. Porter, *The First Queen.*
154. Edwards, *Mary I.*
155. Whitelock, *Princess, Bastard, Queen.*
156. Ibid.
157. Loades, *Mary Tudor.*
158. Porter, *The First Queen.*
159. Letters and Papers, Foreign and Domestic, of the Reign of Henry VIII, Vol. VI, XXI (1882–1920).
160. Appleyard, C. B., Cruz, M. L., & Hernandez, S., 'The Role of Stress in the Pathophysiology of Endometriosis', *Fertility and Sterility*, 2008, 90(Suppl), S35–S36. https://doi.org/10.1016/j.fertnstert.2008.07.1113.
161. Tariverdian, N., *et al.*, 'Neuroendocrine-Immune Disequilibrium and Endometriosis', *Journal of Psychosomatic Research*, 2007, 62(6), pp. 687–692. https://doi.org/10.1016/j.jpsychores.2007.03.008.
162. Ibid.
163. Whitelock, *Princess, Bastard, Queen.*
164. Loades, *Mary Tudor.*
165. Wriothesley, *A Chronicle of England.*
166. Whitelock, *Princess, Bastard, Queen.*
167. Ibid.
168. Ibid.
169. Ibid.
170. Loades, *Mary Tudor.*
171. Edwards, John, *Mary I England's Catholic Queen* (Yale University Press, 2011).
172. Edwards, *Mary I.*
173. Ibid.

174. Ibid.
175. Ibid.
176. 'The Queen's quickening: The phantom pregnancies of Mary I', *Hektoen International*, January 11, 2022.
177. Whitelock, *Princess, Bastard, Queen.*
178. Ibid.
179. Edwards, *Mary I.*
180. 'The Queen's quickening: The phantom pregnancies of Mary I', *Hektoen International*, January 11, 2022.
181. Whitelock, *Princess, Bastard, Queen.*
182. Ibid.
183. 'Endometriosis and Ovarian Cancer', *Journal of Ovarian Research*, 2020, 13(1), pp. 1–10. https://doi.org/10.1186/s13048-020-00637-1.
184. 'Stress and the HPA Axis: Role in Chronic Disease', *Endocrine Reviews*, 2016, 37(5), pp. 557–598. https://doi.org/10.1210/er.2016-1013.
185. 'The Queen's quickening: The phantom pregnancies of Mary I', *Hektoen International*, January 11, 2022.
186. Ibid.
187. 'Endometrial Cancer: Risk Factors and Clinical Features', *Journal of Women's Health*, 2019, 28(4), pp. 456–462.
188. 'Endometriosis and Ovarian Cancer', *Journal of Ovarian Research*, 2020, 13(1), pp. 1–10. https://doi.org/10.1186/s13048-020-00637-1.
189. Edwards, *Mary I.*
190. 'Endometriosis and Ovarian Cancer', *Journal of Ovarian Research*, 2020, 13(1), pp. 1–10. https://doi.org/10.1186/s13048-020-00637-1.
191. Ibid.
192. 'Endometrial Cancer: Risk Factors and Clinical Features', *Journal of Women's Health*, 2019, 28(4), pp. 456–462.

Chapter 6

193. James, Susan, *Catherine Parr: Henry VIII's Last Love* (Stroud: History Press, 2009).
194. Porter, Linda, Katherine the Queen: The Remarkable Life of Katherine Parr, the Last Wife of Henry VIII (New York: St. Martin's Press, 2010).

195. Mueller, Janel (ed.), *Katherine Parr: Complete Works and Correspondence* (Chicago: University of Chicago Press, 2011).
196. Starkey, *Six Wives.*
197. Lindsey, Karen. *Divorced, Beheaded, Survived: A Feminist Reinterpretation of the Wives of Henry VIII* (Reading, MA: Addison-Wesley, 1995).
198. Porter, *Katherine the Queen.*
199. James, *Catherine Parr.*
200. Ibid.
201. Starkey, *Six Wives*.
202. Porter, *Katherine the Queen.*
203. Starkey, *Six Wives.*
204. Porter, *Katherine the Queen.*
205. Ibid.
206. James, *Catherine Parr.*
207. Ibid.
208. Mueller, Janel, ed. *Katherine Parr: Complete Works and Correspondence.* Chicago: University of Chicago Press, 2011.
209. James, *Catherine Parr.*
210. Ibid.
211. Mueller, *Katherine Parr.*
212. James, *Catherine Parr.*
213. Norton, Elizabeth. *The Temptation of Elizabeth Tudor, Elizabeth l, Thomas Seymour, and the Making of a Virgin Queen* (Pegasus Books, 2016).
214. Ibid.
215. Porter, *Katherine the Queen.*
216. Parr, Catherine, 'Letter to Thomas Seymour, June 16, 1548', in Mueller, Janel (ed.), *Katherine Parr: Complete Works and Correspondence* (Chicago: University of Chicago Press, 2011), pp. 171–172.

Chapter 7

217. Wier, Alison. *Mistress of the Monarchy: The Life of Katherine Swynford, Duchess of Lancaster* (Random House, 2009).
218. Ibid.

219. Jones, Dan. *The Plantagenets: The Warrior Kings and Queens Who Made England* (Penguin Books, 2012).
220. Wier, *Mistress of the Monarchy.*
221. Ibid.
222. Ibid.
223. Ibid.
224. Norton, Elizabeth, *Mistress to Henry VIII: Bessie Blount* (Amberley Publishing, 2011).
225. Murphy, Beverly A., *The Bastard Prince: Henry's Lost Son* (The History Press, 2001).
226. Ibid.
227. Ibid.
228. Ibid.
229. Weir, Alison, *Mary Boleyn, Mistress of Kings* (Ballantine Books, 2011).
230. Ibid.
231. Ibid.
232. Ibid.

Chapter 8

233. Briggs, R., *Witches and Neighbors: The Social and Cultural Context of European Witchcraft* (Viking Penguin, 1996).
234. Green, Monica H., *Making Women's Medicine Masculine: The Rise of Male Authority in Pre-Modern Gynaecology* (Oxford: Oxford University Press, 2008).
235. Green, Monica H., 'Conversing with the Minority: Relations Among Christian, Jewish, and Muslim Women in the High Middle Ages', *Journal of Medieval History* 34 (2008).
236. Ibid.
237. Ibid.
238. Ibid.
239. Ibid.
240. Ibid.
241. Ibid.
242. Green, Monica, *The Art of Midwifery, Early Modern Midwives in Europe* (Routledge, 2005).

243. Whaley, Leigh, *Women and the Practice of Medical Care in Early Modern Europe*, 1400–1800 (Basingstoke: Palgrave Macmillan, 2011).
244. Green, *The Art of Midwifery.*
245. Whaley, *Women and the Practice of Medical Care.*
246. Ibid.
247. Green, *Making Women's Medicine Masculine.*
248. Green, Monica H., '*Conversing with the Minority: Relations Among Christian, Jewish, and Muslim Women in the High Middle Ages', Journal of Medieval History* 34 (2008).
249. Schlegelmilch, S., 'The Midwives of 17th century Tübingen', *Medizin, Gesellschaft und Geschichte*, 2005.
250. Ibid.
251. Ibid.
252. Ibid.
253. Green, *Making Women's Medicine Masculine.*
254. Roper, Linda, *Witch Craze: Terror and Fantasy in Baroque Germany* (Yale University Press, 2004).
255. Schlegelmilch, S., 'The Midwives of 17th century Tübingen', *Medizin, Gesellschaft und Geschichte*, 2005.
256. Whaley, *Women and the Practice of Medical Care.*
257. Roper, *Witch Craze.*
258. Ibid.
259. Ibid.
260. Ibid.
261. Ibid.
262. Ibid.
263. Ibid.
264. Ibid.